© **Copyright 2020 - All rights reserved.**

The content contained within this book may not be reproduced, duplicated or transmitted without direct written permission from the author or the publisher.

Under no circumstances will any blame or legal responsibility be held against the publisher, or author, for any damages, reparation, or monetary loss due to the information contained within this book, either directly or indirectly.

Legal Notice:
This book is copyright protected. It is only for personal use. You cannot amend, distribute, sell, use, quote or paraphrase any part, or the content within this book, without the consent of the author or publisher.

Disclaimer Notice:
Please note the information contained within this document is for educational and entertainment purposes only. All effort has been executed to present accurate, up to date, reliable, complete information. No warranties of any kind are declared or implied. Readers acknowledge that the author is not engaged in the rendering of legal, financial, medical or professional advice. The content within this book has been derived from various sources. Please consult a licensed professional before attempting any techniques outlined in this book.

By reading this document, the reader agrees that under no circumstances is the author responsible for any losses, direct or indirect, that are incurred as a result of the use of the information contained within this document, including, but not limited to, errors, omissions, or inaccuracies.

Table of Contents

INTRODUCTION ....

CHAPTER 1: COMPULSIVE EATING EXPLAINED 6

CHAPTER 2: OBESITY DEVELOPMENT 22

CHAPTER 3: INVESTIGATION AND ACKNOWLEDGEMENT 40

CHAPTER 4: SELF-LOVE JOURNEY 56

CHAPTER 5: ANCIENT KNOWLEDGE AND ASSISTANCE 72

CHAPTER 6: LET'S GET PHYSICAL 88

CHAPTER 7: SET THE BALL ROLLING 104

CHAPTER 8: PREPARATION FOR ALTERATION 119

CHAPTER 9: DETOXIFYING YOUR TEMPLE 134

CHAPTER 10: THE NURTURING DIET 148

CHAPTER 11: BONUS EXAMPLES 167

CONCLUSION 169

REFERENCES 172

Introduction

Christian Larson once said, "Believe in yourself and all that you are. Know that there is something inside you that's greater than any obstacle." I cannot agree more with this. Obesity, overeating, binge eating, and our obsession with food are merely obstacles in the way of reaching our full potential.

Ask yourself if you're happy with the way you live. We are often confined to our bedroom or couch most days because we don't have the energy left to move our bodies. We find ourselves gasping for air when we cry out for the fresh air that surrounds us but our body resists. Are you truly happy with the way you feel? We become deeply depressed when we no longer find joy in the activities we once loved. We would rather hide in our homes and avoid the judgment we believe is inevitable from our peers.

Do you really find comfort in being a type two diabetic in your glorious youth? The thought of not being able to eat the products we once loved because they can send us into a vicious hypoglycemic attack is certainly not something we want anymore. The pain over our heart is even less welcome in our lives. How can we forget the discomfort of being immobile on some or all the days we live on this planet? Don't you yearn for the socialization you thrived in when you were a kid? Can you remember the days your friend list included everyone on the playground and running was part of every minute of the day? We welcome boredom into our lives when we're restricted by our movements and feasible activities. Boredom and loneliness often walk hand in hand and take no prisoners.

Even when we have a partner there's deep-seated anger, guilt, and sadness for not being able to join them in hobbies and interests. An overwhelming lack of confidence in ourselves creeps up before we know it. Compulsive overeating reaches into the particles in every aspect of our lives. It grabs our happiness and taunts our physical strength. It plays games with our emotional wellbeing and mocks our self-worth.

Things don't need to be this way anymore. I can see an ignition rekindling the embers that have burned inside you before. They're stroking the passion and need for change that can redirect your life permanently. There's something about the word "permanently" that gets my juices flowing. I've introduced myself before and you're aware that I suffered for years with tragic and devastating health conditions caused by my inability to find the right answer to my questions. The truth is actually that I suffered three major and life-threatening eating disorders that began in my teenage years and persisted well into my adult life. I admit that I didn't see the problem at first and it was the influence of other people who altered the first two disorders. My mother was threatened with social workers when I was in high school, and as a child, people were there to guide me.

Unfortunately, they misguided me and led me to the doorstep of another disorder. My second compulsive behavior was kept a secret, or so I believed. My husband eventually figured it out and tried aimlessly to help me. The disorder had dug its roots deep into my mind after years of practice. My loved ones approached the problem in the worst possible way; they attempted to control me like Geppetto controlled his puppets. That only encouraged me to become ultimately covert in my behavior.

Unfortunately, this behavior took many aspects of my health permanently and could have killed me at any moment. It wasn't until life threw me lemons, faster than I could turn them into lemonade, that I turned to compulsive overeating behaviors because I gave up on life. My weight and health took a drastic beating before one photo changed my life. It finally brought me to my knees and made me realize that I would die young if changes weren't made immediately. Doctors had tried to convince me for years that my health was critically dancing with the grim reaper, but the photo is what ultimately pushed me over the edge.

It's been years since I last binged on anything, and after various failed diets, I found one combined technique that worked because it targeted every reason for my disorder. The main focus of this book is to aim at removing compulsive overeating and allow you to live a wholesome life you desire, but I'll give you a short intro on my other disorders because I know this approach can work for any eating disorder. Everything that happens in our lives stems from a deeper place within us, and I've learned to use a perfect balance of science (Murphy et al., 2010) and ancient practices (Kristeller & Wolever, 2011) to reset my brain after years of brainwashing myself.

I spent time choosing the right pre-diet and diet to supplement my change and provide me with the comfort of products I can relate to. There's nothing worse than having to change your personal taste to remove this problem from your life. I learned about the physiological changes that take place and the reason I became so sick from my choices. There are methods of halting the progress of these ailments and giving yourself a fair chance in life again. You'll learn about altering your habits, thoughts, behaviors, and embedded beliefs in such a way that you don't fear the change anymore. I've found ways of caressing my emotions and living with the fact that I'm not alone. This pandemic has struck the modern world like a nuclear explosion.

That's why I choose to share my findings and personal success with you. I've fine-tuned the process of removing these habits from my life and implementing new habits I enjoy that will prevent me from ever slipping back to where I was. I can't promise you a permanent change, but I can guarantee that this is the best shot you have to become a healthy, happy individual again.

I know how sensitive I was about my choices when I sat in the same boat as you. Therefore, I've used a precise language and method to convey my message. Please do not feel offended at any word I speak because the only way to tackle an extremely sensitive issue is by using an engaging and entertaining language. I wish all the people who tried to help me, in the beginning, used this tactic because I find it easier to listen to someone who grabs my attention.

Now, I want you to take my envisioned hand and walk through this with me because it's best done as a team. Remember that someone does care because I care about the place you're in now.

Chapter 1: Compulsive Eating Explained

There's often a misconception of compulsive eating and I aim to remove any misinterpretations of the condition. A variety of disorders exist and there are numerous warning signs to look out for if you're trying to help yourself or someone you care about. The comprehensive details on symptoms that accompany eating disorders will be expanded so that you can diagnose yourself with the malady because it's often difficult to recognize our faults.

The Definition of Compulsive Eating

Where do we start when we're faced with a problem we deny? The beginning of this journey lies within recognizing what the problem is. You can't face an issue when you deny the existence of it. This remains true with every aspect of life. Someone who drinks alcoholic beverages excessively is often blinded by their perception. They develop tunnel vision and see no error in their decisions. They often cannot see the impact drinking has on their lives until it reaches astronomical significance and ravages their life to shreds. Just as alcohol impairs people, so does food and lifestyle. The food we consume is frequently overlooked, along with the snags it cultivates.

Life was so much simpler in ancient times. Heck, it was even effortless in the early 1900s. We weren't surrounded by endless temptations and food to console ourselves. What happened to the days where grass-fed animal and vegetable products were eaten as staple foods? Now we consume large laboratory-produced T-bone steaks at lunch and drown our cereal with refined sugar and pasteurized milk. We drink coffee out of habit and find solace in stuffing our faces when we're confronted with challenges in life. Come on, I know you've heard the phrase "comfort food" before. You know what I'm talking about. As humans, we have found comfort in eating to overcome the trials we meet. I'm not immune to this habit myself as I've succumbed to the same persuasion before. However, when I found out what defined this eating disorder, my vision changed, and I began looking for answers.

How does one describe compulsive eating? I want you to focus on the word "compulsive." The description which immediately comes to mind is revealing in itself. Compulsive means to have an irresistible urge which stems deep within you. Your urge overwhelms your senses and brain to create an irrefutable delusion. "Irresistible" is another keyword because you can't resist something that creates an overpowering desire inside of you. This influential impulse convinces you that what you desire is compulsory. It tricks your mind into altering a basic desire into something you strongly believe is needed for the likes of your survival and happiness. It becomes your only desire when you experience this impulse. Compulsive behavior is dangerous, to say the least.

When this impulse is combined with the vast array of foods, healthy and unhealthy, it explodes into a detrimental behavior of overeating. Compulsive overeating portrays itself as someone who consumes colossal amounts of food or calories that aren't perceived as normal. It doesn't necessarily mean the person eats their food in five minutes. Overeating or binge eating can also present itself as someone eating more food in two hours than someone else would eat over two or three meals throughout the day.

If you look at someone and their portion of food is substantially different from yours, it could indicate that you're overeating. In some cases, the portion may resemble yours in size but yours is smothered in gravy and three variants of sauces with a stack of fries that reach for the heavens. Ask yourself one question: Are you able to finish a large pack of potato chips and a jumbo soda in five minutes without feeling satisfied? Do you eat for flavor or is it an absolute necessity for you to finish your plate of food? Think about the last time you were so stuffed that you placed leftovers in the fridge for the following morning. There may be a problem if you can't remember a time you didn't finish your meal.

Nevertheless, compulsive eating is a behavior common in many serious eating disorders. It's not an eating disorder on its own but it's a behavior that accompanies potentially life-threatening eating disorders. It describes the action of eating uncontrollably and having no brakes. The person will find themselves eating until they become physically uncomfortable and their button is about to pop. They may continue eating until they become sick in some instances. They lose the ability to recognize when they're satisfied and fail to slam on the brakes on the train of consumption.

This behavioral disorder results in you feeling out of control in your own body. It can intensify to a point where regulation is long lost. Sufferers can be enticed to eat after smelling something delectable, even though they've just eaten. They become a zombie who's lost all impulse control and the mere sight, smell, and even audio stimuli can activate the cravings like a zombie craves the flesh of another person. Compulsive eating zombies might start eating to a point where their upper abdomen extends, and they experience pain in their lower chest from the pressure on their diaphragm.

Compulsive eating contains impulse control distortions. However, it also consists of obsession with food, weight, and physique. An obsession creates another insalubrious train smash with desire. Therefore, having a compulsive eating distortion can be defined as having an obsession too.

What Kind Are You?

Compulsive eating has various stages and some people are in the beginning stages and others are in a more serious condition. To determine what phase you may be entering, we need to discuss the various kinds that exist. Six different eating disorders are recognized as mental health conditions, some of which relate to some form of obsession or compulsive behavior according to Healthline (Petre, 2019). The information is compiled by Dietician Alina Petre who graduated with a master's degree in sports nutrition in the United Kingdom. I am, however, going to focus on the disorders which relate to our discussion only.

There are a few rare eating disorders I'd like to discuss first. The first of which is called night eating disorder. I believe this is common in our discussion. This describes people who wake up in the middle of the night and binge on a few calories before they go back to sleep. Another interesting thing is a condition called orthorexia. It's yet to be classified as an eating disorder, however, this describes someone obsessed with healthy food again. This is the opposite of what we're discussing but I wanted to mention it because you'll learn about balance soon enough. There's no point in tipping the scales so that the other side is weighed down excessively in the light.

There's one condition that's rather disturbing and it's called rumination disorder. This condition defines someone obsessed with the compulsive behavior of regurgitating their food as sheep do. They chew their food and even swallow it, but as a scary twist of events, they voluntarily bring their food up to graze on it a second time. The physical process resembles acid reflux and not purging or vomiting. Anyway, this disturbs me deeply and I just wanted to share the information. It's not completely relevant to my guide but allows you to see that you're not crazy. There are disorders out there that challenge common sense. To put your mind at ease, this condition can be improved with the information in this book too.

Pica is another condition that isn't our main focus, but it does contain hints of impulsive behavior. This is when someone irresistibly craves substances that aren't classified as food. It can include cravings for laundry detergent, chalk, soap, paper, dirt, ice cubes, hair, pebbles, cloth, and wool, among other things. We won't pay much attention to this condition because it's common among pregnant women without impulse control, children needing essential vitamins, and severe mental disabilities.

Now I'll focus on the three eating disorders that hurt my health excessively because I want you to understand them. Anorexia contains strong elements of obsessive behavior even though it doesn't relate to our topic of conversation. This describes someone obsessed with their weight and physique, no matter how tremendously skinny they may be, you can't convince them otherwise. Their obsession isn't directly related to food and that's why they're not on our target list. This was my first obsession and it began in my teenage years.

We now come to the two disorders that deserve our spotlight in this book: bulimia and binge eating disorder (BED). Compulsive overeating is common among these conditions and I'll give you a breakdown of these disorders.

Binge eating disorder is one of the most common eating distortions in the United States, according to the National Center for Biotechnology Information. The article included the fact that BED is more prevalent among older individuals and males (Frédérique et al., 2012). Binge eating disorder describes someone who binges on exorbitant amounts of food in short periods of time and uses no means to correct the high-calorie intake. Doesn't this sound familiar? This is one condition we'll focus on because people with BED frequently gain exorbitant amounts of weight. If the condition is targeted early enough, the weight gain can be reduced and halted. Binge eating disorder sufferers have little to no control over their impulsive behavior.

Bulimia nervosa also catches our attention because it's another compulsive behavior disorder. According to Alina, bulimia is more prominent amongst women rather than men. People with bulimia enter an obsessive binging stage where they lose all control over the amount of food they eat in a confined space of time. Bulimia sufferers often find themselves full to a painful position and they love targeting food they would normally avoid in their daily lives. They can binge on any food though; it's not just limited to avoided foods. Once this person is uncomfortably full, they purge their meal to return their gut to comfort and attempt to shake the calories they've consumed. A purge can include excessive exercise, laxatives, diuretics, fasting, enema usage, and forceful vomiting. Bulimic people are usually in a normal weight range even though they believe they're overweight.

Both BED and bulimia nervosa can be life-threatening if left untreated. If you suffer from an eating disorder, I suggest you keep reading to dive into the details of your problem before you resolve it. I suffered from anorexia, followed by bulimia, and finally BED I've conveniently compiled a chart to show you the probability of developing certain eating disorders using information from the National Eating Disorder Organization.

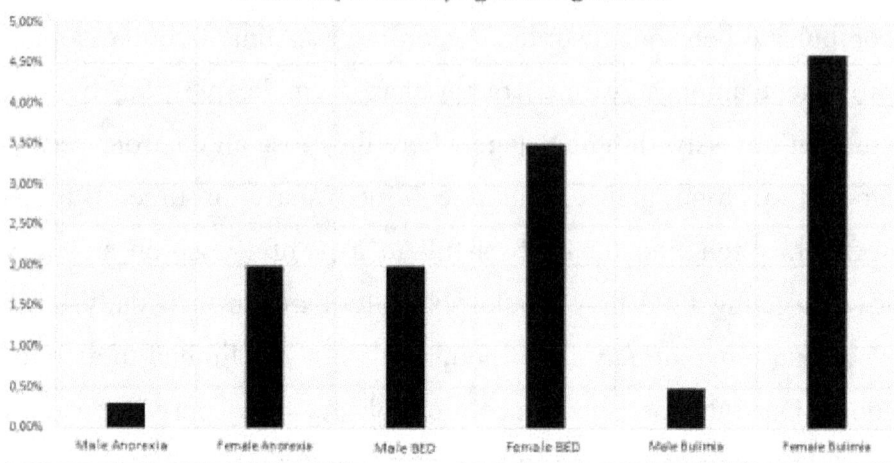

Common Symptoms

I know that I've touched a nerve here and you want to know more. You might have suffered the same chain of events I did before you reached obesity. Nevertheless, there are symptoms associated with compulsive overeating and some of them can indicate a specific disorder. I'm going to guide you through identifying worrisome symptoms, but an accurate diagnosis should be specified by a doctor, nutrition specialist, or a therapist. You'll understand why a therapist gets involved in later chapters. I aim to help someone who suffers from compulsive overeating in general and my advice will pertain to that. This section is written to help you identify potential symptoms related to a specific condition, but if you want a genuine diagnosis, that can't be achieved yourself.

Typical symptoms tied to compulsive overeating, in general, include a variety of tell-tale signs. If you can relate to even one or two of these signs, you're most likely suffering from this impulsive alien. Someone who overeats impulsively will eat amounts that are larger than what someone else would consider rational. They could eat at a speed which puts Michael Schumacher to shame (Schumacher is a retired formula one driver who was contracted by the likes of Ferrari). On the other hand, you could eat at the speed in which David Hasselhoff moves in his infamous slow-motion Baywatch program. Unfortunately, people who eat with persistent buffering can result in never finding an end. They commonly eat non-stop throughout the day.

Eating until their bubble is about to burst is another easily identifiable symptom. They eat past a state of suffice and frequently indulge in consumption when they're not even hungry. They could begin eating out of boredom or to soothe any emotional disturbance. Feelings of guilt and shame drive them to eat alone because they're afraid of judgment on the size of their portion or embarrassed by their manner of consumption. They inevitably feel guilty, depressed, and even disgusted in themselves after binge eating. They find themselves divulging in the temptation in the middle of the night when the world is asleep. The most frightening tribute is when they begin hiding their food or eating in secrecy.

In 1999, there was a movie called The Spy Who Shagged Me and it starred Mike Myers as Austin Powers. It was a huge hit and I personally loved the Austin Powers movies, as corny as they were. However, Myers doubled as another character in this specific rendition who tugs at my heartstrings. The character was called "fat bastard" for comedic purposes but one line from the movie is true. Fat bastard lies on the bed, in his sumo outfit, indulging in food, and says, "I eat because I'm sad and I'm sad because I eat." There's an undeniable truth in his words and another symptom you can identify eating disorders with is the irrefutable connection between your emotions and eating. Someone who impulsively divulges in excessive amounts of food will become depressed about their obsession and, in turn, the depression will worsen the problem. Look out for these signs as well because they play a large role in your behavior. I'll discuss emotions and the connection in detail later. The bottom line is that emotional distress after eating a meal is a definite sign of consumption issues.

On a more serious note, there are additional symptoms linked to the conditions mentioned in the previous section. Someone who suffers from BED may feel out of control when they eat. The second symptom is when someone excessively overeats and has no accountability for their behavior. They recognize a problem, but they don't care about the consequences. They use no form of purging to supplement their behavior and go about life gaining weight and increasing the risk to their health. Don't get me wrong, purging is extremely dangerous to your health as well.

When it comes to bulimia nervosa, there's also no perceived ability to regulate their actions and a sense of ill management exists. Additional symptoms can include a severe fear of gaining weight even though their body mass index is normal, a brutally impaired self-esteem about themselves, and purging. Their purging habits can include any of the rituals discussed in the previous section.

You may be embracing a corrupt eating habit if any of the symptoms are prevalent at least once a week for three months or more. If you're experiencing these symptoms like a new addition to your life, you should step up immediately. The sooner you correct the problem, the easier the task will be. The good news is that overeaters are usually aware of their symptoms and that itself is another symptom. They acknowledge that their eating habits are abnormal.

Warning Signs of a Compulsive Eater

Unfortunately, some people will live in denial even though others can admit their shortcomings. Psychology will help us understand the reason why some people refuse to admit that they have a problem, but in the meantime, I want to share some warning signs you can look out for in a loved one who may have fallen prey. My purpose in this guide is to help someone overcome a terrifying nutrition disability but that goes for someone who may be trying to help a friend as well. Not one person in this world is immune to falling into the trap of impulsive eating and it can grab a hold of your sister, uncle, friend, mother, or son. What do you need to know in addition to the symptoms we've discussed to recognize a potentially harmful condition lingering in your loved one?

The National Institute of Mental Health claims that three percent of teenagers are inflicted by this and four percent of adults at any given time (Kay, 2016). Those figures speak for themselves. Assessing yourself is simple but evaluating a loved one can be difficult. They'll hide most of their symptoms and you'll need to look out for signs they can't conceal. The fact is that people who haven't reached the stage of asking for help often have an advanced stage of eating disorder before it's recognized by loved ones. This places their health at increased risk and therefore I want to delve into the details before it gets out of hand. They may not be as lucky as I was in defeating death. Please take a moment to identify any of these habits to understand how advanced your possible condition has progressed itself.

The first sign is an obsession with food, diet, and physique. Does the person endlessly talk about losing weight or going on a diet? Have conversations ultimately veered in the same direction over and over? Someone who discusses an issue progressively and non-stop is displaying signs of an obsession. When you love something you can't stop talking about it, right? This obsession can extend to exercise too. The person may become angered by their inability to exercise and you notice no increase in their calorie intake to level the playing field with their physical activity.

The second sign can indicate their lack of control. By this, I mean something different from what we've already discussed. An unhealthy eater may become agitated or angry because they can't control the recipe and the ingredients it entails. They could even lose their temper if dinner plans change and they obsessively felt the irresistible urge to eat at the local buffet tonight because it's an excuse to "pig out." They'll make excuses about how they starved themselves all day to save space for dinner. Please note that these excuses are sometimes false.

Obvious signs to watch out for are irregular behaviors during and after meals. Does your loved one often disappear after eating? They claim they have a small bladder and need to run to the bathroom. They also become uncomfortable when other people are present. They may use words like, "I'm a shy eater." This may seem insignificant, but you should observe any odd traditions closely. They've never been particular about the order in which they eat their food but now suddenly they've adopted a new culture where starch must be consumed before vegetables and meat. This helps when they purge because they need heavier food to assist the lighter food to expel itself from their body.

Another sign is inexplicable mood changes. Someone who was always Daphne of the group has suddenly become morbidly depressed and agitated. Daphne's smile is synonymously known for describing someone who's always joyful and wants to hug the world. However, a sudden shift in any emotional direction can indicate a problem with your loved one. Drastic mood changes in teenagers are common with eating disorders.

Another warning sign can be quite visible. The person may show extreme fluctuations in their energy levels. This can go either way and they can remind you of a bear that needs to hibernate or someone who can fragment the world's energy crisis with their endless amounts of energy that originate from thin air. Does your loved one look constantly exhausted even though they haven't exerted themselves? Do they have a new hyperactive energy that can't be pinned down?

The final warning to scan for can lie within their physical symptoms. Is their weight fluctuating aggressively? This is easier to identify when you know their habits and lifestyle. All of a sudden their weight changes and they've gained 20 pounds with no reason visible. Other physical signs to watch for include decaying teeth and a change in their breath odor.

Before you move on to the next chapter, I want you to process the information you've read. Do you recognize these worrisome signs in yourself or a loved one at risk? Find the strength you have within you to defeat denial and become critical of yourself or your loved one. Overeating compulsively is a dangerous game and I'm going to share everything I've learned with you.

Chapter 2: Obesity Development

The main focus in this guide is your binge eating disorder and obesity, so I'll circle back around to the matter at hand. Life has developed over the decades and so has our waist sizes. Although modern life offers many beneficial advancements in food, leisure, and technological advancement, it has had a devastating impact on American citizens' health. What do doctors consider a health risk and what does overeating do to us physiologically? The impact extends beyond our bodies and into our minds. How do these physical changes affect our future wellbeing?

A Growing Social Issue

The extent of damage caused by obesity and BED are connected to our lives being simplified. Just the fact that you live in a first-world country has already added a contributor to your list. The epidemic hasn't impacted developing countries as significantly as the United States because poverty is ripe in those regions. Even though they too are entering the modern world, they're behind on the obesity scale linked to Americans. Let's take one example I've learned from a friend in South Africa recently. She admits that South Africa has the obesity epidemic itself. However, they watch the developed countries and manage to learn from some mistakes and take inspiration from others. She insists that the spectrum of influence from other countries, unfortunately, doesn't always resonate through government and policy.

In 2016, a new South African legislature was passed to implement a forced tax on sugar. The hope was that adding a 20% tax on sugar products will deter consumers from purchasing vast amounts of refined sugar products. The bill was passed in 2018 and since then sugar prices escalated substantially. I was pleased to hear this because if a developing country is changing laws to curb the effects of obesity, it means they have jumped on board after seeing the epidemic hit their shores.

It's not only what we consume that has changed our lives. I'll refer back to another movie that was popular because it was a collaborative effort between Disney and Pixar in 2008. I'm sure you've heard of *Wall-E*. Even animation touches on the truth of what's happening in the world and depicted it in a movie that opened eyes. Wall-E was a mechanical robot built with a purpose in mind. He was tasked with cleaning the world while humans were floating about in space. My point doesn't refer to Wall-E though; I want to discuss the humans who were stuck on Axiom. This was the gliding spaceship that housed Earth's humans for 700 years while they waited for Earth to be inhabitable again.

When the movie focuses on the people in the ship, as amusing as it may have been to some, it's disturbing to others. Axiom is filled with morbidly obese men, women, and children because their lives have been lived for them. They maintained no physical exertion and were fed an array of modern and fast foods. They were so overweight that they couldn't walk anymore and were hovered about on robotic chairs. Technology became the inevitable companion of these people and their eyes were so glued to screens that they didn't even socialize anymore. Half the time they would glide right past someone while talking to them on their futuristic mobile devices.

This is what's happening to the world in real life. It's not a series of animated motions but a genuine threat to our lives. Technology encourages our lazy lifestyles and the convenience thereof has made us forget what it's like to live in the physical and mental presence. Virtual reality is one I'd like to target because it allows someone to slip into a simulated scenario where they can hike into the mountains. What happened to hike up the damn mountain? The fresh air on your face, the smell of nature, and the genuine fatigue that follows are all dissipating.

Besides modern advances, food has become as lazy as we have. Fast food is especially a bad apple. No, it was far too inconvenient to take a drive and watch the world around you on your way to dinner. Fast food kicked it up a notch when the delivery system came into play. Fast-food chains and restaurants are capitalizing on faster delivery times, larger portions, and free giveaways to boost their business. They increase their profits by substituting organic and fresh ingredients for others that keep piling on the pounds. The next time you order a triple chicken burger drenched in processed sauces and accompanied by enough fries to feed an army, ask yourself one question: Is this real chicken and potatoes? That's some food for thought.

It doesn't stop there though. Our food is being grown in laboratories now because the population is exploding, and the resources can't support the increase for much longer. Stem cells are used to grow beef burgers in a lab. I mean that's seriously ridiculous! If you don't do something to prevent modernization from consuming you, you've already lost the battle. My rant is over now, but it grinds me when people deny the role that modern society plays.

BMI: What Is Considered Obese?

According to the world population review, the United States is 16th on the list of highest obesity rates in the world. This is shocking when you consider how many countries were evaluated and many of the countries above us are islands. The countries that outweigh us, pun intended, are American Samoa, Tokelau, Nauru, Cook Islands, Palau, Marshall Islands, Tuvalu, Niue, Tonga, Samoa, Kiribati, Micronesia, Aruba, Kuwait, and the Cayman Islands.

If we look at the population as of 2019, the only country that has a vast population is Kuwait. They have over four million people and all the other places range between 1,600 people and 200,000. This shows a frightening truth because these countries have higher obesity percentages among their tiny populations. The United States recorded over 329 million residents in 2019. Even Mexico, which has over 127 million people, ranks lower on the list (Most Obese Countries Population, 2019).

I've compiled a graph below to compare the United States to other well-known countries. The figures are based on a percentage of the population whose BMI is over 30.

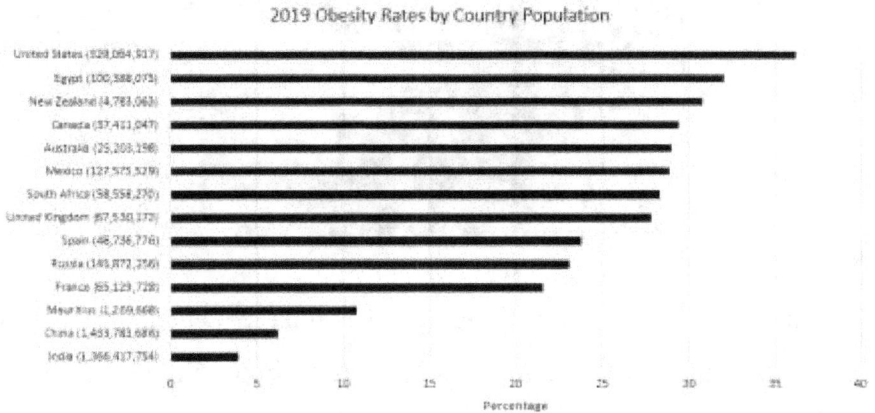

If the sheer numbers don't shake the foundations of your mind, you need some more convincing. The statistics were based solely on the population number versus the body mass index of the people. Body mass index, or BMI, is what doctors use to tell you whether you need to lose weight. Fortunately, you don't need to visit your practitioner to know what's normal. A BMI is a calculation of your body mass or weight and your height to attain a value. This value indicates whether you're underweight, normal, overweight, obese, or morbidly obese.

HEIGHT	WEIGHT (POUNDS)															
	100	110	120	130	140	150	160	170	180	190	200	210	220	230	240	250
5'0"	20	21	23	25	27	29	31	33	35	37	39	41	43	45	47	49
5'1"	19	21	23	25	26	28	30	32	34	36	38	40	42	43	45	47
5'2"	18	20	22	24	26	27	29	31	33	35	37	38	40	42	44	46
5'3"	18	19	21	23	25	27	28	30	32	34	35	37	39	41	43	44
5'4"	17	19	21	22	24	26	27	29	31	33	34	36	38	39	41	43
5'5"	17	18	20	22	23	25	27	28	30	32	33	35	37	38	40	42
5'6"	16	18	19	21	23	24	26	27	29	31	32	34	36	37	39	40
5'7"	16	17	19	20	22	23	25	27	28	30	31	33	34	36	38	39
5'8"	15	17	18	20	21	23	24	26	27	29	30	32	33	35	36	38
5'9"	15	16	18	19	21	22	24	25	27	28	30	31	32	34	35	37
6'0"	14	16	17	19	20	22	23	24	26	27	29	30	32	33	34	36
6'1"	14	15	17	18	20	21	22	24	25	26	27	28	30	32	33	35
6'2"	14	15	16	18	19	20	22	23	24	26	27	28	30	31	33	34
6'3"	13	15	16	17	18	20	21	22	24	25	26	28	29	30	32	33
6'4"	13	14	15	17	18	19	21	22	23	24	26	27	28	29	31	32
6'5"	12	14	15	16	17	19	20	21	22	24	25	26	27	28	30	31
6'6"	12	13	15	16	17	18	19	21	22	23	24	26	27	28	29	30

It's rather easy to work it out yourself if you have a calculator handy that is capable of calculating a square root function. Divide your weight in pounds by your height in inches squared. Then, you multiply the result by 703 and round it off to the nearest decimal amount. The result you see will give you a figure like 22.7, and this is your BMI. If your weight is 192 pounds and four ounces, you can convert this to a decimal factor again. One pound is 16 ounces, so four ounces will equate to 0.25 pounds.

There's a standard rule that most dieticians and doctors will abide by when understanding someone's range classification. If your BMI lies below 18.5, you're considered underweight. If your BMI is between 18.5 and 25, you're considered a perfect and healthy weight. When your BMI ranges between 25 and 30, you are overweight. When your BMI exceeds 30, you're classified as obese. A BMI above 40 is considered morbidly obese.

Look at the chart to get an overview of BMI by weight and height. The highlighted numbers indicate a healthy weight range, the numbers to the left indicate an underweight person, and the numbers to the right move into overweight and obese.

Hormonal Imbalance: What Happens Physiologically?

The human body is an intricate design that houses delicate processes. Hormones are one of the physiological changes that take place in your body when you experience compulsive overeating. I'm going to attempt to use plain language to describe the process that takes place when you suffer from an eating disorder or binge eating.

There's one gland in your brain called the hypothalamus and it's located below the thalamus and above the pituitary gland. It sits on the bottom surface of your brain and is an almond-sized organ of the limbic system. Your limbic system is accountable for memory and emotion regulation. The amygdala and hippocampus are connected to the limbic system as well. Nevertheless, the hypothalamus itself is responsible for your sleep cycle, your hunger tuition, and behavior, among other roles.

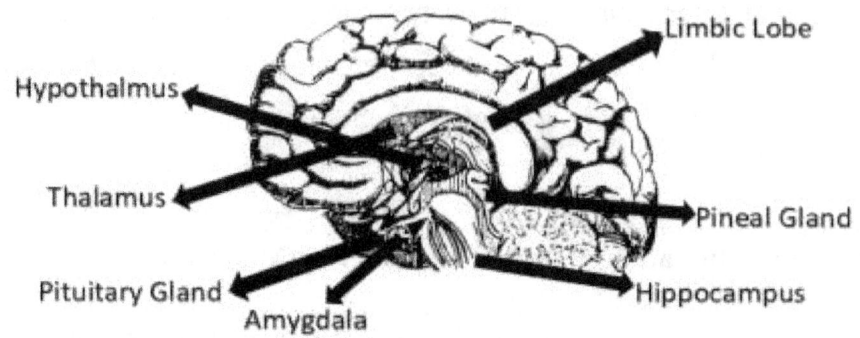

The second team player I want to discuss is called the endocrine system. This describes a messaging network that extends to every part of your body, including all organs and glands. Chemical messages travel through this network to specific organs and instruct them to release chemicals in your bloodstream. The hypothalamus uses this network to send messages and so do other glands such as your thyroid and adrenal glands. Hormones encourage growth, keep your metabolism intact, and even orchestrate your reproductive system. The endocrine system maintains a perfect balance in your body. But this balance can be shoved off track when an eating disorder plays ball.

Some hormonal changes that take place have been extensively studied because this subject has intrigued scientists for decades. There's evidence to suggest that binge eating can cause a dysfunction in your limbic system and your hypothalamus doesn't know when to signal your satiety anymore. When the hormone involved with satiety stops functioning, you're constantly hungry. It leads the way to a vicious cycle of not knowing when you're full and you continue to falsely believe you're hungry.

Your hypothalamus enters an overdrive state and misfires infrequent signals to your adrenal glands to produce cortisol. Cortisol is another hormone and it regulates stress responses in your body. An increase in this hormone or an irregular production can lead to increased heart rate and blood pressure. The terror doesn't stop there either. Cortisol encourages the production of insulin in bulk by raising blood sugar levels during an imitation phase. When your insulin increases, your body craves sugars and unhealthy fats to replenish it, leading to excessive weight gain.

This inevitable avalanche of hormonal disaster continues when it restricts the production of the leptin hormone. Leptin regulates energy consumption in the small intestine and prevents you from getting hungry when you're satisfied. It also reduces fat in your body. The cascading effect continues when the morphological structure collapses. This is the organism that branches and maintains relationships between organisms in your body. Studies show an increase in visceral fat in your abdomen after this collapse.

Your limbic system fails to produce enough of the estrogen hormone and that leads to sexual and reproductive issues. Women can suffer dry, burning, and itching vaginas as they would with menopause. Testosterone levels decrease and men struggle with sexual desire, sperm production, and various other issues with the prostate and testicles (Warren, 2011).

Numerous other hormonal changes take place and that can fill a book on its own. For now, the following are the changes I'll share with you.

Psychological Blockages

With your limbic system under attack, there are psychological problems that will ensue. Some problems will follow, and other problems can be to blame. How could this overeating disorder have manifested itself in you?

Eating disorders are commonly associated with other mental conditions such as depression, social anxiety disorder (SAD), post-traumatic stress disorder (PTSD), general anxiety disorder (GAD), and obsessive-compulsive disorder (OCD). There's no surprise on the last of the supplementary conditions. Obsessive-compulsive disorder is a mental disorder that describes someone obsessive and compulsive in their behavior. They always aim to be perfect, whether it's in their hygiene, their persona, their achievements, or an obsessive repetition in the pursuit of perfection.

A perfectionist isn't quite the same though. I can think of Nicolas Cage who acted as an OCD sufferer in *Matchstick Men*. He displayed repetitive behavior, and if something wasn't in his control, he couldn't emotionally handle it. He would experience a tic where his facial muscles would spasm. Cage is a brilliant actor for his role in this movie among many others.

Anyway, someone who suffers from these conditions lacks coping mechanisms, also known as coping skills deficit. As soon as they lose control over a situation, their default method of coping lies within distorted eating behaviors. They obsess over correcting the issue with dangerous habits, whether it's overeating or purging. You can call this a tic of sorts. Their impulse takes over when they face emotional distress and they enter their alternative reality of being able to control their weight in bulimia or expose themselves to food and a certain lifestyle to cope with the changes. Depressed people are frequently in a gloomy mood and social anxiety encourages someone to fear judgment from people because of the way they look or the food they eat. I have to admit, I suffer from OCD. I've been diagnosed; it's not a phantom thought. Therefore, I can tell you that my tics included unhealthy eating behavior.

PTSD sufferers look for comfort in extreme measures to remove the constant replay of traumatic events in their minds. This could even include someone who can't overcome the death of their loved one. This is another condition I've embraced after losing someone and witnessing a traumatic event. General anxiety disorder is when someone gains an extreme fear of losing control. This could include a wide variety of fears and must be diagnosed by a professional. However, these conditions have all been linked to eating disorders in psychology. Two in every three people with an eating disorder commonly suffer from some form of anxiety, especially OCD (Cowden & Gans, 2019). All the conditions mentioned in this section are subcategories of anxiety, except for depression which simulates a grieving process. Depression is the process of grieving change in your life. It can include losing a loved one, your job, a friendship, or even moving from one city to another. Depression leaves you yearning for something you once had.

I want to share one psychological trait with you. I suffered from relatively low self-esteem as a child. Most days I would feel worthless, unloved, and unwanted. As any child does, I sought attention. I began looking in the wrong places because I wasn't receiving it at home. My parents were robotic and moved about on autopilot. I can't remember any shows of affection from them.

Unfortunately, my coping skills deficit derived from depression and OCD, lead me to seek attention with my peers at school. However, I thought I wasn't attractive enough, and over my younger teenage years, I became a walking skeleton. This had the opposite effect and boys were repulsed by my bony structure. Girls made fun of me and I became physically sick. I could stand in front of the mirror when I weighed the same as an eight-year-old child, yet I would still see flab everywhere. I was obsessively in denial.

My school therapist saw a problem in my malnourishment, and I was placed on a strict diet at school and home. This is how my bulimia began because I continued seeing someone who was fat, even though people were disgusted in my scrawny physique. The bulimia persisted for years and eventually crossed over to a point where I stopped caring during my married years. My husband's persistence was admirable but unfortunately, he didn't focus on all the problems. My purging ways flew out the window, but my binge eating didn't when my first true life stress hit me. I lost my mother, step-father, and my husband's work placed immense pressure on us for years. I lived in fear from his ties to judicial uniform and our lives were targeted at home when I was personally attacked. I had to comfort my emotional damage somehow. When I became obese, my depression and social anxiety deepened because I was self-disgusted and disappointed in myself. Sadly, this never made me stop. I suffered from morbid obesity for years, along with my depression and anxiety, before I learned the secrets of correcting the entire problem.

The bottom line is that psychology and eating disorders go hand in hand. It's a vicious cycle that never ends unless you end it. One of the two always influences the other. I advise you to put your embarrassment aside and seek psychological help in addition to the physical and mental changes you're going to implement yourself.

The Devastating Consequences

There are physical consequences to eating disorders as well. The problem isn't only mental and emotional. I'm going to focus on the physical conditions related to bulimia and binge eating disorder specifically because I've suffered one too many myself.

Bulimia nervosa comes with a string of health risks involved. It starts with dehydration and a sore throat. The act of purging through vomiting is particularly violent on your system and can go beyond pain when you rupture tissue in your digestive tract. It's common to suffer from water retention in your arms, legs, and even face when you purge regularly. Your teeth decay from the stomach acids that pass, and digestive issues persist, including constipation, diarrhea, and chronic bowel obstructions when your colon becomes spastic. You're frequently over exhausted and the constant insulin manipulation will result in long-term damage to your organs.

Your electrolytes are minerals essential to your body's proper functioning, and when these electrical impulses throughout your body malfunction, it can result in damage to your heart. It will start with heart arrhythmias and can lead to cardiac arrest in some people. That's a general overview of bulimia perpetuation. I experienced most of them and suffer from congestive heart failure today that finds its roots in electrolyte imbalances combined with my cholesterol and obesity later on.

Binge eating disorder has its own set of complications. One of them is all too familiar with you and that's obesity. There are more sinister complexities that often elude you. You may be aware of some of them.

Your skin and hair will suffer when your skin becomes dry and your hair becomes fine and brittle. An increase in sugar intake leads to acne and so does dairy products for some people. All the carbohydrates you're consuming will prompt your body to burn excess energy to digest the food and you'll fall into a sleeping beauty phase, without the beauty of course. There will be an uncomfortable pattern of heartburn, indigestion, frequent diarrhea, acid reflux, and stomach cramps. Eating excessive amounts of food will go one step further than discomfort and stretching your stomach can lead to a rupture. The medical terms consistent with this are gastric dilation and gastric perforation. Irritable bowel syndrome will knock on your door as it did mine.

BED is also linked to high blood pressure that relates to its own problems. Diabetes is another common denominator in binge eating and something to take note of is that you don't need to be obese to start suffering these consequences. Although obesity leads to issues with cholesterol that clogs your arteries and can also create cardiac issues. If you indulge in high fat binging, you can suffer from gout. Gout is one painful form of arthritis when there's an excess of uric acid in your bloodstream. This forms crystals in joints, typically in-between your toes that makes walking unpleasant.

The stereotype of people eating themselves into oblivion prevents you from seeking help. Besides future health complications, you affect your financial stability, work security, interpersonal relationships, quality of life, and life expectancy. Please acknowledge that binge eating leads to severe complications just as much as anorexia does. Never allow the thought to enter your mind that people are just going to judge you. I've created a chart of the standardized mortality ratio (SMR) for binge eating disorder. This is gobsmacking because it means that one in five deaths in the United States is related to health conditions caused by obesity, specifically BED.

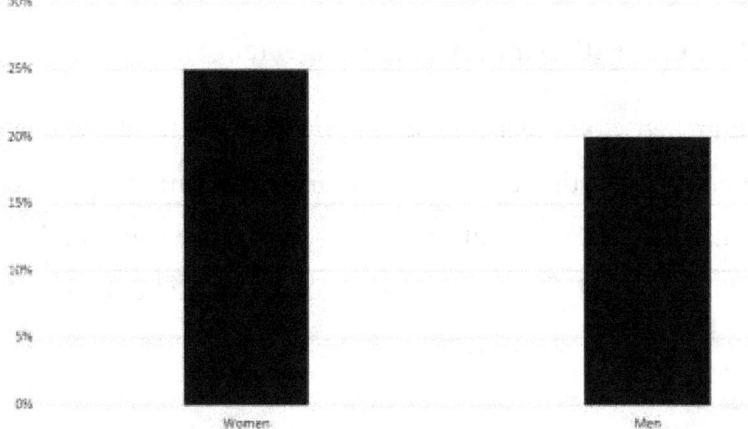

Chapter 3: Investigation and Acknowledgement

You're frightened after learning about the changes taking place. Now you need to investigate the contributors in your life: dietary and environmental factors. Your habitual vices play a role and you doubt there's a route forward. Does one give up or do you take the bull by the horns? I know you're not going to give up.

Placing Your Diet Under the Microscope

Investigating your diet is the first step before you can understand what's making you ill. You want to expose the monster that deprives you of living the life you want to live by opening a can of worms. I hope you don't intentionally open a can of worms. I've seen weirder fetishes than worms when it comes to food.

Silkworms are a popular delicacy in China and the fat mopane worm is commonly eaten in Zambia and Zimbabwe. The formal name is Gonimbrasia Belina and it's the caterpillar that grows into an Emperor Moth. They get their name from the mopane leaves they eat. People describe them as crunchy on the outside and there's a burst of juice when you bite into the worm. The Democratic Republic of Congo offers tourists a delicacy of crickets that provide the same crunch when you bite down on them. Cambodians have a fetish with eating tarantula spiders and China prides itself in the thousand-year-old eggs. These eggs are not a millennium-old egg but rather preserved over a few months. The Chinese use a concoction of clay, quicklime, and ash to preserve them and they resemble a hardboiled egg from a horror movie. The yolk often turns a slimy black and the white becomes a dark translucent jelly. They smell like ammonia mixed with sulfur but taste amazing. Many people advise that you hold your breath as you eat them to prevent yourself from succumbing to the rotten smell.

Anyway, back to identifying your food habits now. Yes, my irrelevant deviation had a point. It was meant to distract you for a moment and brew deep nausea within you before we speak of food. I have my unconventional methods of removing my mind from tempting food and I've shared one with you briefly. Good luck with overcoming the stew of disgusting thoughts I've installed in your mind. I learned this trick many years ago and it's never failed me once.

Moving on, only you can recognize the foods for what they are. I want you to think about the symptoms you've read and try and connect them to food that's made you feel the way I described in the previous chapter. Has your fat and oil-drenched fried chicken from the Colonel caused you heartburn? Are you thinking about the inability to stay awake during your Netflix marathon last night when you ate two donuts and three packs of skittles? You were alert for the first episode of the *Santa Clarita Diet*, but you can't recall an episode after the first? The fact that the sitcom didn't displace your desire for eating is another item to add to your list. Your body went into a sugar high before you crashed. Did you find yourself holding your chest as your heart palpitations left you wide-eyed after that bowl of popcorn you besieged in salt? Keep panning through every notable experience you've had that relates to any food you've consumed.

The first exercise I'll give you is to correlate any foods and food types you've eaten before you experienced the symptoms listed in the first chapter. This helps the process of acknowledging the foods you divulge in that lead to your concerns. You're welcome to add any foods that make you feel depressed and any other emotions that derive from your diet. Spend a few days devising your list of food triggers and keep them handy for the advice I'll present soon enough. This exercise doesn't necessarily relate to your dietary changes on their own. It will help you recognize symptoms you've overlooked before.

Changes in Your Life

The next exercise I need you to complete is one that pinpoints your emotional and psychological sources. You have core beliefs inside of you and those have rooted somewhere in a collection of experiences you survived in the distant or recent past. Core beliefs are the very idea inside of you that direct your thought patterns and emotional responses. I've learned some valuable manipulation techniques from a therapeutic method known as cognitive behavior therapy or CBT. This therapy has existed for decades now and finds its inspiration in ancient methodology and philosophy.

I've spent weeks delving into CBT with a therapist and it has helped me change the way I think. I'll use a summarized definition of the technique so that you can understand where I'm going. Cognitive behavior therapy is brief but hands-on psychotherapy used to alter people's thinking patterns and behavior. It digs deep into the source of your problems before it provides you with the tools to change your patterns permanently. I find it highly inspirational in changing the way I see myself and the world around me.

I've found a valuable insight into core beliefs during therapy. These beliefs don't just pop up on their own. They grow with us when we're children and can even develop in relationships throughout our lives. Events and experiences have changed the way we believe in something. See the chart to understand how various risk factors predispose us to eating disorders.

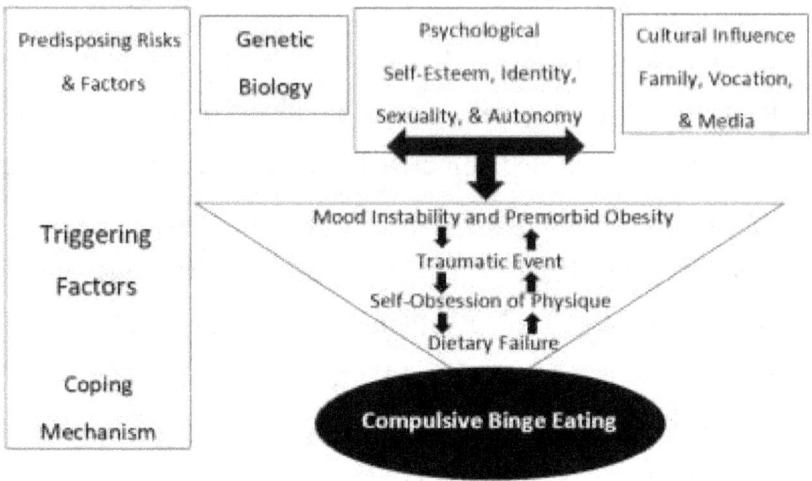

I've touched on this subject in the psychological aspect of compulsive overeating and I'll elaborate further now. When you're a child who grew up in a household where love didn't exist, you're predisposed to believe this with every molecule inside your body. It's not just the act of your parents failing to tell you how much they love you, but other factors too. Perhaps, your parents never had a loving relationship of their own or no one showed any affection for another person in the home whatsoever. Your family may have made you feel unlovable from the start.

Now you have become an adult and you seek the same relationships you've grown up with. Do you know how people often say that your wife resembles your mother? Well, that has something to do with your core beliefs. You're convinced that this is reality and the world works this way, so you're attracted to someone who thinks and feels the same. Sadly, you fail to recognize the automatic thoughts that follow because deep inside you believe that you're unlovable.

The same concept applies to your eating habits and overall perception of health. You grew up in a house where every family member was obese, and they all ate five turkey legs dunked in a honey glaze for lunch. Obesity and overeating have become an obscure reality. Forget about the emotional aspect for a moment and think about the first time you ate dinner out at the buffet. Did people stare at you as you chipped away at the corn like a woodchipper? Did you not perceive your eating habits as perfectly normal before you began noticing the emotional trauma linked to this scenario? You might have believed that these people were damn rude for staring. I've experienced this on several occasions.

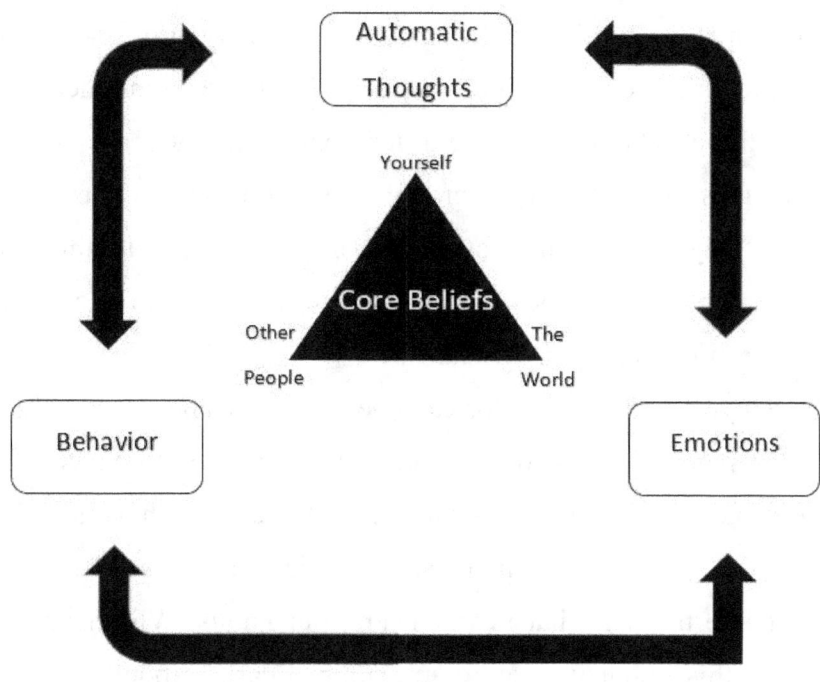

This is one concept of a distorted reality or cognitive distortion. There's another side that frequents eating disorders, especially when your core belief system appears reasonable. Maybe you grew up in a home where nutrition was considered a daily factor in the equation and a trauma in your later life has led to your dysfunctional belief system. This is where emotions come in from the start. You become wary of your environment and the people that fill its space. You know that your newfound belief doesn't match your childhood belief but you're so depressed that it doesn't matter.

You walk into Walmart and purchase five gallons of carbonated sugar-filled soda and enough food to feed a small village. The food consists of chocolates, potato crisps, three cheeseburgers, a full loaf of white bread, ten slices of cheese, and a roll of processed ham. You're preparing for your binge session tonight and the moment you arrive at the checkout, you have a deep paranoia that grabs hold of you. All these thoughts rush through your mind and suddenly the checkout lady knows all about your binge session. Nothing can convince you that she doesn't. You enter a panic mode and words leave your mouth in a nonsensical flow.

I've given you one example for each belief failure and I want you to think about the moments you *may* have experienced before recording any possible traumas or deep-seated core beliefs that have allowed this behavior to continue. The reason for this exercise is to help you acknowledge the pain that lies beneath your habits. Why have you given into this impulsive nature and stopped caring about yourself? Keep your notes aside for your future reference and you can add to them as you recover from this disorder.

Identifying Habits That Aid the Process

The next exercise I'll share with you is to help you acknowledge any lifestyle habits that perpetuate your disorder. What is food in your opinion? How does food help you escape the reality of any traumas, fears, and emotional disturbances? I can give you an answer because it's simple. Food addiction is merely a coping mechanism to find comfort from the issues in your life that taunt you. Unfortunately, there are coping strategies that synonymously accompany eating disorders.

Substance abuse is one of these parallel coping skills we adopt. I'm not saying that every single person who battles binge eating disorder will suffer from substance abuse, but it can happen. According to the *Eating Recovery Center*, approximately half of people who suffer from eating conditions are known to abuse one or other substance (Lewaniak, 2016). These escape techniques may help you forget your problems for the immediate future. However, they can wreak further havoc on your system.

Alcohol abuse, in particular, has allowed me to escape reality for a few hours. The only problem was that I'd wake up the next morning with a hammering migraine and all my problems will ogle me on a magnified level. Not to mention the health risks that go hand in hand with alcoholism. Alcohol combined with binge eating over an extended period can lead to potentially life-threatening damage to your organs. Alcohol has played a role in obesity and will also halt weight loss when it spikes your glucose levels.

Prescription and non-prescription drug abuse are other common problems because you begin using excessive amounts of sleep aids when you fail to sleep with restless legs at night. Your heartburn keeps you awake until the early hours of every morning and your only emission from this is higher schedule drugs. Focus on finding these inconceivable vices that hinder your progress. Smoking is another vice that raises your blood pressure further and adds to your respiratory problems, especially in obese people. Do you want to sleep with that offensive and noisy mask over your face as Mike does in the sitcom *Mike and Molly*? If you're already using one of these devices, you can certainly improve your breathing abilities by following my advice. However, don't deviate from using your device without your doctor's consent.

Vices that you can consume are not the only target of this step. You can think back to my rant about the modern world and all its technological contributors. Anything you find yourself relying on is considered a vice. If you couldn't dare imagine getting off the couch to change the channel, then your vice lies within the convenience of a remote control. Yes, you can add that to your list.

One of the first things on my list involved removing all the applications on my mobile phone that helped me be as lazy as I had become. I was able to order food on easily accessible apps to be delivered straight to my door when I was morbidly obese. I never had to drive to collect my toxic fast food, and so many of these franchises offer free delivery to gain more clients now. Do these buffoons realize what they're doing to us? Anyway, the same advice goes for any application that changes your channels, switches your lights on and off, and any games that simulate real-life activities.

Identify any "convenience processors" in your life and record them on your list. Remember to keep speed in mind too. Do you purchase all these microwave meals at month's end? Does your freezer contain multiple precooked meals that you can pop into the microwave for 30 seconds? All you have to do is pierce a few holes in the cling film cover and read the instructions on heat setting and time. Yes, I've hit the nail on the head again. There's nothing I won't cover because I've been through it all.

One touchy subject you can acknowledge is for people who are morbidly obese and use mobility scooters. Do you own one? How often have your feet touched the ground since you bought it? It's just another mechanical robot that makes your life noxiously simpler. You'll see where I'm headed with this soon so don't submit to confusion and wonder why I'm asking you to identify each of these modern vices.

Research on Viable Reversal

Before I reveal my plan of action for you, the first of many, I want to show you the evidence behind my perceived madness.

An article was published in the *Journal of Consulting and Clinical Psychology* in 2011 (Grilo et al., 2011). The article covered a vast range of clinical trials and meta-analysis gathered over the years. One study specifically wanted to test the possibility of cognitive behavior therapy on obese patients with binge eating disorder through behavioral weight loss and cognitive restructuring. One hundred and twenty-five obese patients with BED were randomly allocated to one of three groups to receive CBT treatment followed by behavioral weight loss (BWL) treatment. Each participant was assessed directly after treatment ended and again at six- and 12-months post-treatment.

The cognitive restructuring resulted in higher remission rates among the evaluations and BWL showed promising decreases in BMI ratios during treatment. Cognitive behavior therapy showed increased viability rather than BWL in the long-term but BWL provided evidence for weight loss as long as treatment continued. In layman's terms, this means that CBT treatment established new thinking patterns and the participants used these new skills to build a future that promised healthier choices. Unfortunately, BWL on its own doesn't achieve long-term results and participants fell back into old habits.

I hope this helps you understand my faith in a treatment that has changed my life. Everything I do is based on inspiration from CBT, along with new habits and lifestyle changes I've gained experience with.

Is This Battle Possible?

It's finally time to reveal my purpose for introducing CBT methodology. The study I shared with you proves one major fact. The reality behind overcoming your malady lies within your mind. Have you heard the phrase "old habits die hard"? Benjamin Franklin was the first person to cite this phrase in 1758. The first evidence of the phrase dates back as far as 1450 according to Gregory Titleman, author of *America's Popular Proverbs and Sayings*. Why has this proverb stood the test of time? I can only think of one reason, and that's the pragmatic answer we all know. People love this saying because it's true.

Please note how the proverb speaks of changing your habits as a challenge. Nowhere does it ever mention impossibility. That alone should answer your question. Of course, change is possible when you use the right tools. Cognitive behavior therapy has been used for decades to alter behavior and habits in people and I spent a lot of time learning how to do that. I've worked collaboratively with a therapist to get the ball rolling. Do you want to know what the best part of this treatment option is? It's the fact that you gain the tools to replace thoughts, habits, behavior, and beliefs yourself. I emphasize the "self" part of that sentence. That's why they call it a short-term therapy because it only teaches you how to do it yourself.

I want to help you change your mental perception and habits by remembering the tools I learned in my therapy. Remember that I'm not a therapist; however, nothing is holding me back from sharing my journey with you while including the methods that worked for me. Changing habits is indeed difficult but you'll use mind restructuring techniques to do it. The circuitry in your brain needs to be rewired and that takes practice. When you're assessing one problem, remember to dig deep into your logical mind to analyze the issue thoroughly. Look at all outcomes, consequences, and potential alternatives. You can even use a moment of pause to accomplish this.

Now that you have your self-assessment of your impulsive and obsessive behavior, I want you to set yourself a goal. This goal can be recorded on multiple sticky notes that you spread around your home and workplace. There's a system I learned to use in CBT when it comes to goal setting and it's called the SMART system. The acronym stands for specific, measurable, achievable, realistic, and timeous. Make sure that each goal you set is detailed and choose specific milestones that have no generalized form. You can set milestones in your goal to measure your progress.

Your goal should be within your capabilities and it should be realistic for your current state. Please don't target a new walking routine every morning when you're bedridden from obesity. You have to start with standing on your feet for a couple of minutes at a time. The final stage is setting the start line in your goal marathon. The SMART system has helped me set multiple goals and my aim has changed over the years. I'll add and remove goals often, depending on environmental and life changes.

Keep your goals close to heart as well because you're likely to succeed if you set them within your comfort zone. When you fail at achieving a milestone, take a step back and analyze the outcome, your thoughts, emotions, and any possible alterations that can make the goal achievable. Don't allow failure on your first or even second attempt to deter you. I can honestly disclose my few failures when aiming for targets that were above my reach at the time. Keep each milestone small. Don't write the first milestone as "lose 50 pounds" or "burn 30 inches of fat around my midsection in two weeks." That's highly improbable and you should consider the little demands first.

Add a sticky note to your refrigerator door and below your shopping list, which reminds you of the consequences of eating three cheeseburgers at once. You can make notes of exactly how it made you feel and even add a reminder of the awful night spent in the bathroom for hours.

Finally, I want to refer back to the method of distraction I used at the beginning of this chapter. I know it was sly to surprise you like that, but distraction is another key aspect of CBT. It's one of the common exercises I used in treatment, and after completion of the collaboration effort, I continued using it. I've simply kicked it up a notch since I began. Google and YouTube have often helped me when I want to remind myself of the visual effects of my previous condition. Okay, this is referred to as exposure therapy in CBT, but I'll find myself searching for some medical video that shows me the inside of an obese person's gut. It has diverted my attention on many occasions.

You can even distract your mind with a completely irrelevant idea. Are you feeling hungry right now? I want to tell you about this amazing creature I saw on the Discovery channel. It was called a sparklemuffin and I've never seen anything more interesting in my life. Australia sure as hell has weird and wonderful creatures but this little spider remains my favorite. It's also commonly called the peacock spider and when you see a picture of one, you'll understand why. It looks like a hairy spider until you see the head. The head resembles an octopus and is as colorful as a peacock's tail feathers. More amazingly, the eyes are attached in a circular form surrounding the oblong head shape. I promise you'll love the little bugger.

And that's how simple distraction is. Work on becoming the master of impromptu thoughts and allow your mind to wander away from the thoughts and emotions that drive you to eat or even food itself. It may be challenging at first. However, with enough practice, you'll become king or queen of impromptu distraction. I consider myself a master of distraction and should join stand-up comedy. I have honed the ability to look at a situation and immediately I have 20 humorous thoughts pop into my head. This is where I want you to be.

Chapter 4: Self-Love Journey

Suffering from a lack of self-worth is probably what caused your dilemma in the first place, no matter how this came about. The beliefs instilled in your mind since childhood have distorted your reflection of who you are. Your relationships have either destroyed you further or encouraged your behavior. You need to replace your connections with those which will improve your life and finally allow you to express your needs truthfully. It's time for you to learn self-love before you continue on this journey.

Self-Esteem Significance

It's true, you'll find it increasingly challenging to promote a different life if you think of yourself as worthless, valueless, and a fat nobody. Your self-worth or confidence in yourself is what drives your decisions in life. It acts as a motivational train that speeds toward a split in the tracks and it can decide which intersection your train will follow. If your motivation is aligned with higher self-worth, it will help you annihilate any obstacles on the tracks gracefully. Your engine will progress full steam ahead toward any goals and aspirations you've set.

You don't believe that you're worth any acknowledgment or reward for your achievements when you have low self-esteem. You also don't have the zooming cart of motivation to reach your destination. Your resilience barrier is down and anything negative that comes your way is just accepted. You don't question anything that you should, even if it doesn't align with rational thinking and you lose the will to keep moving forward. Challenges become inadvertently insurmountable and the only thought in your mind is to quit. Well, guess what? Quitters never win! I won't provide you with the motivation to quit.

The problem you face is that you have no idea what high self-esteem feels like. It's an alien concept to you and it's difficult to understand something you've never had or encountered. If you're an unlucky bugger who believes that you've never seen this extra-terrestrial, please take a moment to consider something you love. It could be a person, a pet, or even a car. I'm going to use a pet as an example. Your dog, which we shall call Duke of Hazzard, has been with you for years. He's an older boy and has a little extra weight himself. How do you feel about Duke? I know you love him deeply and couldn't imagine life without him. He lies at the end of your bed every night and brushes his hair against your toes. His slobbering mouth wets your feet because he has a short muzzle. You love Duke so much that these things all seem insignificant.

You are his world and he may be yours too. He couldn't possibly survive without you. You fill his bowl every morning with dry food and hand him a dog biscuit every night before lights out. He's been a loyal canine and has crept his way deep into your heart. Okay, now you have a sense of your feelings towards Duke. Someone who has high self-esteem would feel this way about themselves. They would care that their heart is failing under the weight of their mass. They'll want their body to be clean and free from burns in the sweaty folds. A confident person radiates with positivity and smells like a freshly powdered baby. You fear for the life and safety of Duke because you can't live without him either. Now you're getting the right picture.

There's another danger and you should be careful not to overbalance your self-worth. No one likes a cocky egotist either and I've dealt with too many of these assholes. I specifically mean smug public speakers who think they've achieved a feat that no one else can. Their delusion makes them believe that they're the only person in the world who lost 75 pounds. Apologies, but I love going into a rant.

You want your persona to come across as humble without actually calling yourself that. Allow yourself credit when credit is due and don't take responsibility for something that wasn't you. When you reach your first milestone, you certainly earned your worth. It doesn't matter how menial it may seem to uneducated people. I've noticed this in eating disorders particularly and someone who hasn't been there has no idea what an accomplishment it is when you haven't indulged in chocolate for the last six days.

I know how large that is, but some people won't. Unfortunately, these people may assume that you're bordering on narcissistic tendencies. Someone who inaccurately thinks you have an overinflated ego will only hurt your self-esteem more. Your loved ones and anyone else who knows the long road you've walked to overcome your challenges will see your pride as plausibly deserved. Balance is key and you'll find it with time. Reaching a healthier and wholesome life after battling emotional turmoil, eating disorders, and being obese is something you may feel proud of in my opinion.

Targeting Your Core Beliefs

Let's discuss some more psychological aspects. Information processing happens when we try and make sense of what happens around us. We observe a situation and immediately our core beliefs interrupt our perception of what we see. Your core beliefs don't only change the way you perceive your worth but the worth of others around you is involved too. Your brain is constantly overwhelmed by high volumes of electrical impulses or information that needs to be processed and the fastest way for you to do this is reverting to what you believe. Your attention shifts to what expectations align with your belief system and often these expectations are beyond realistic.

I refer to an example of someone who grew up in a home filled with dysfunctional eating behavior. Your core belief is telling you that being overweight and eating compulsively is normal and within your expectations. Now, let's add some spice to the recipe and stage a scene where you sit down with familiar faces. I'll call these people new acquaintances. The first time you met them, it was at an all you can eat pizzeria and there wasn't a person at the table who didn't have at least five slices of true American style pizza. This has only added to your core expectations because first impressions leave a lasting effect on us.

Now you meet them in a steakhouse that's famous for a food challenge you know about and instantly you ask them if they'll also be having the two-pound T-bone challenge. The challenge consists of two pounds of meat, a triple portion of fries, and a half a gallon of sugary soda that has to be consumed in less than 30 minutes. Suddenly, everyone stares at you as though you're from another planet. You can't blame them because you've automatically associated them with your first impression dangerously combined with your core beliefs. Your interpretation was false when you assumed and expected these people to act the same way as the time you met. You've even failed to notice that one of the ladies is as skinny as a stick insect. This is an obscure example of overblown self-esteem.

On the other hand, someone with low self-esteem will persistently play down their accomplishments and damage their self-worth more with each failure to recognize them. Challenge your belief system by questioning your thoughts. Do you jump to conclusions when you eat a regular slice of lemon meringue? You've gone without eating treats for three weeks now and you've just spoiled yourself to one reasonable slice. You haven't made a habit of it. You're only rewarding yourself for three weeks of following your new lifestyle. A reward is needed in behavior therapy because you want to know how it feels to change a traditional habit. You're using another CBT technique called operant conditioning, or positive reinforcement as most of us know it. It doesn't matter if you intentionally rewarded yourself or it was a slip up when you ordered a meal. Allow yourself the reward either way, as long as you refrain from entering another binge eating cycle. Psychiatrist Stephen Gans from Massachusetts General Hospital supports behavior modification and it can apply to any situation or problem (Cherry & Gans, 2019).

Using subtle positive reinforcement over a prolonged period will encourage the new beliefs in you. Remove that thought in your mind right now because you're not weak. When you've gone weeks without an old habit that derived from your skewered reality and belief system, you're most welcome to reward yourself. I would use clothing as a reward rather than sweet treats though. Buy yourself a new shirt or some spunky underwear when you've stuck to the plan for four weeks straight. I have a closet full of clothes to remind me how spectacular I am.

Learning to Love Yourself

Loving yourself is the way you permanently shift your self-esteem in the correct direction. Do you remember Duke? Great, now I'll guide you to loving yourself appropriately and without obsessing over yourself. You should find the same love for yourself as you do for Duke.

The first step is to learn to find comfort in loneliness. Begin planning activities that you love and do them alone. You don't need to rely on someone else to be happy because every person has various hobbies and desires. The moment you depend on someone else to make you happy is the moment you fail to be content with your own choices. Your opinion matters to you and that's all that counts. This was a major turning point for me, and I grew comfortable with being by myself rather quickly when I realized how great it feels.

This may be difficult at first, but I also suggest that you remove yourself from any comfort zone and step into the world of curiosity. This enhances many aspects, and by trying new things you can learn just how competent you are. Have you ever wanted to play an instrument? This is something you can do even before you burn the fat that makes you feel undesirable. Open yourself to new possibilities with talents you might never have acknowledged before. Your current situation and physique don't need to hold you back, and people, including yourself, will automatically overlook your body shape when you're hitting those ivory keys passionately and reaching Elton John tones. I've seen some incredible musicians who are overweight, and it makes no difference to their talent. Opera tells another story because overweight people have used their lung capacity to vibrate those notes to a whole new level.

Forgiveness is the next step in loving yourself. No one in the world is without fault and the moment you learn to forgive the mistakes you've made is the moment you win at this game. Journaling your emotions and thoughts will give you insight into how strong you truly are. You'll look back at obstacles that made you feel weak and worthless and realize that you've used new skills to cope with them. You've found your David and finally defeated Goliath.

Stop being hard on yourself and allow yourself a breather once in a while. You can take a trip to the mountains to breathe in fresh air when you feel overwhelmed. Don't push your fragile mind and body into submission and be kind to your limits. There comes a time when you must place your needs ahead of others and this is the subsequent step in your progress. It's as simple as practicing the word "no." You don't have to please every Tom, Dick, and Harry. If you decide your weight must reach a BMI score of 27, then so be it. Don't allow Adolf Hitler's mentality to dictate your progress.

Open yourself to challenges, and if you've spent the last two years perfecting a new design for a unique dress, have a little faith in yourself and send that email out. You may not be able to wear this gorgeous outfit now but the day you see it on someone's body, your heart will skip a beat and every low thought you've had of yourself will dissipate. Until you challenge yourself in life, you won't know what you're capable of achieving and you'll never know how good it feels when your dress is the next hit on the runway. Schrödinger's cat is a typical assumption in quantum mechanics. If a cat is stuck in a box, it is both alive and dead until you open the box indefinitely and find out. Go ahead and open the box to see if your cat is alive. If the poor cat has succumbed to death, move on with your head held high and open the next box.

Trust is one delicate issue and to reach the goals you've set for your journey to a healthier life, you need focused trust in your abilities. Never question a decision you make unless it falls by the irrational wayside. The deeper your trust becomes, the easier you'll trust other people.

The final stage is stating the obvious because you can't love yourself if you don't take care of yourself. If you've spent years as a bulimic, your teeth have their own story to tell. Why should you accept this? Book an appointment at the dentist and have your teeth fixed. You won't believe how confident I was after having a dental makeover. That alone brought me to tears and I looked in the mirror to see a beautiful smile staring back at me. The only thing I could see before my makeover was a fat and disgusting shape in my reflection. People often forget that beauty has various definitions. Someone who's overweight but carries themselves well in public acts with poise and looks like an advert for Colgate always permeates confidence. An even radiance of self-esteem is gorgeous on its own.

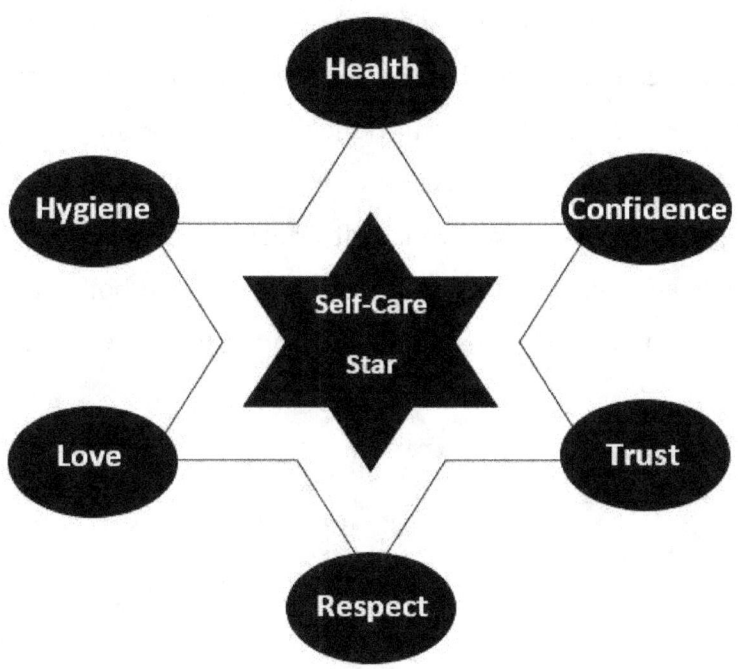

Relationship Focus

My focus on relationships is another two-way street. Low self-esteem can chase your loved ones away and being in a bad relationship can beat yours down with a baseball bat. Your objective is to remove any irregular and harmful relationships and replace them with mutually loving relationships because you deserve it as much as the next person does. Low self-worth can drive your partner away, especially intimate or romantic partners. It doesn't discriminate against other relationships either.

You become insecure and attach yourself inappropriately to the other person, smothering them and making them wish to run for the hills when your self-esteem is low. Your partner may display this attachment toward you and keep you from fulfilling your potential. Obsessive behavior yoyos between you and you want to control your partner or vice versa. Unfortunately, relationships have no boundaries when insecurities are involved. This mother goose bondage will break down your self-esteem and leave you feeling unlovable and make you resent your partner. You'll both either have separation anxiety or never be able to stand in the same room.

Jealousy is another critical component of insecurity. Both of you will become overly possessive of each other because the green-eyed monster is lurking about. There will be an unbalanced level of neediness, and when the potentially obese party becomes too clingy, they can hit the ground hard when a partner leaves them. As this control-orientated relationship continues, one party will feel the need to ask permission for any decisions that shouldn't necessarily be mutual. Suspicion can brew between you and a complete lack of communication can break you down because your mind is free to wander about the realm of fantasy.

The possibility of cheating and lies creep into your relationship and you know that's a recipe for emotional anguish. On the other hand, your suspicion may be unsubstantiated, and your relationship falls due to false accusations. Someone with low self-esteem could even lose interest in the relationship themselves for no reason. Whereas someone with healthy self-esteem would focus on using their relationship to enhance their life. Unfortunately, if you don't love yourself, your relationship will struggle under the weight of these insecurities among others and dissolve.

As much as you believe that you're better off without your partner or friend, entering deep loneliness isn't advised in this case. However, if your partner is undermining you and using these insecurities against you or they have their own insecurities, dump them or divorce them. Two people who love each other, whether as friends or lovers, should love each other and themselves. I like the word partners because being with someone is a partnership. There are no 50/50 partnerships because if my partner gave me 50% of him, I would shove him out the door of a moving train. I want 100% of his efforts and I am responsible for giving him the same.

When you see any red flags and you feel as though your partner is the reason you feel no value in yourself, I suggest you take my advice on the moving train, figuratively of course. The kind of relationship you want to be in when boosting your self-esteem is one that benefits both of you. There should always be a perfect balance of love and compassion between you. Communication should flow freely and if you're on this journey, you need a partner and friend that will support you through it all. You don't deserve any less and you can't be around someone who enables the lifestyle that hurt you in the first place. If your partner needs this journey as much as you do, encourage them and be their pillar of strength.

Voice Your Truth and Your Needs

Finding your voice is the final stage of giving you a quick boost in loving yourself. I've started using these daily and they give me the courage to speak my truth. I would voice these affirmations in the privacy of my home, and I sounded like a shy schoolgirl who's been confronted by her teacher when I began. My voice grew louder and so did my confidence as I continued my practice. Have you ever heard someone say that you speak negativity or positivity over your life? Affirmations are even used in CBT therapy and ancient philosophies because hearing the vibrational sounds of your voice has a genuine impact.

It's one simple technique to overpower negative thoughts and any self-sabotaging considerations in your mind. I'll share a few with you that you can start with. You'll learn to voice your affirmations according to your truth and needs as you grow more confident. Spend five minutes every morning standing in front of the mirror so that you can see your face and make eye contact with yourself as you speak these words. Repeat each affirmation at least five times and try and use the powerful voice that lies deep inside you. I know it's there just as much as you do.

I am a unique person and I acknowledge my existence as being different from everyone else's.

I have a need inside me just as everyone else does and that need screams for self-love.

I choose to become a ray of optimistic sunlight that radiates through my own life, as well as others.

I choose to place a priority on my urgent health needs and eradicate any habits that impact me negatively.

The world doesn't have preferences and my problems are experienced by other people too.

My disorder doesn't discriminate against age, ethnicity, or culture.

I am perfectly capable of digging deep and finding the true purpose of my life.

I refuse to allow depressive thoughts to enter my body because I am in full control.

I no longer see a challenge in meeting new faces and judgment is only in my mind.

I accept the person I am because I have a unique set of talents.

I am the author of my own story and no one can influence my direction.

I acknowledge inspiration growing inside of me and I aim to inspire others.

I deserve compassion and respect from people, and they deserve mine.

I am strong enough to face any fears that cross my path.

I look forward to the new person I will become on this journey.

The power of change exists in me and it's up to me to activate it now.

There's nothing more important in my life than my own decisions and opinions.

I can see an improvement in my physique, health, and mental acuity daily.

I naturally speak my confidence, and nothing can get me down anymore.

My passion for life, love, and the future grows stronger every day.

Chapter 5: Ancient Knowledge and Assistance

Rewiring your brain is the starting line in your marathon, but where does it come from? How do these ancient techniques alter something as intricate as the mind? Mindfulness is one method that's survived for centuries and will endure for many more. This chapter will provide a meditative session that targets compulsive eating to move you one step closer to a wholesome life.

A Brief History

Mediation is used worldwide for a vast array of issues and spiritual purposes. Don't concern yourself with the spiritual aspect of it because we're focusing on the healing side of it. It's up to you if you ever want to dive into the spiritual world. Nevertheless, there's a history that accompanies meditative practices that goes back to a time before Jesus was born.

Do you know why the practice has existed for centuries? It works like all the practices that persist and that's why it lasted. It may have been honed to perfection over time and seen many variations for different needs but the principles of it have remained the same. Before I tell you about what it does for you, I want to give you a brief history of it.

Mindfulness has made its way from the east to the west. Many historians believe that it originates in Hinduism, but it had its part in Buddhism and even Christianity. Hinduism gathers the benefit of credit because it's considered the oldest religion to exist that's still widely practiced today. An interesting fact is that Hinduism wasn't called that in its origin years and was Westernized as what we know it today by the British who refer to it as a single entity religion from the Vedic period in India. It was in fact, not a single form of religion in its beginning years.

The traditions practiced for what we know today began 4000 years ago and continued gaining momentum during the Vedic period. This is when Gautama Buddha influenced the philosophy himself during his travels through the Indus Valley. There are mentions in these ancient scriptures that indicate mindfulness. It was used to gain access to higher knowledge and being closer to Gods during this era. Hindu followers practiced techniques during this period that resemble modern-day meditation and even yogic poses.

Mindfulness was further honed by Buddhism when Gautama was born. He was a thinker and grew up under the influence of Hinduism in the region of Nepal. Both religions and philosophies center themselves on a Sanskrit word "dharma." The translation of this word has been debated to vast extents, but it means a way of life more than a religion. It describes a harmonious way of life that allows you to live in alignment with the natural order of the universal presence around you. There's a sense of give and take and flowing with the direction the universe takes you.

In Gautama's lifetime, the philosophy began splitting into various segments already and was followed by numerous schools of thought. Some of these include Theravada Buddhism, Zen Buddhism, and Mahayana Buddhism. Zen Buddhism, being a more Westernized modern version.

If we take a huge leap forward in history, you can look at someone like Jon Kabat-Zinn who's responsible for creating the Center for Mindfulness at the University of Massachusetts Medical School. Kabat-Zinn continued with his interest and developed the Oasis Institute for Mindfulness-Based Professional Education and Training. He didn't stop there either because he is the founder of the well-known Mindfulness-Based Stress Reduction (MBSR) program which is widely used to conduct clinical trials today. This eight-week program was aimed at reducing stress and anxiety and includes meditative and mindful practices (Selva, 2019).

Thich Nhat Hanh, another name synonymous with modern mindfulness, influenced and taught Kabat-Zinn as one of the many Buddhist philosophers involved in his enlightenment. This is when eastern philosophy clashed with western science and the widely known practice of mindfulness spread like a virus throughout the world. It was after this that mindfulness became an influential player in CBT treatment. Mindfulness-Based Cognitive Therapy (MBCT) rose to the challenge and proved effective in many mental and emotional dysfunctions.

A meta-analysis was published on Springerlink in 2019 that assessed multiple studies conducted on the treatment of eating disorders after implementing mindfulness techniques in psychology (Turgon et al., 2019). The efficacy of mindfulness-based programs was conducted on specific issues such as BMI alteration, emotional adjustment, body discontent, and negative effects that receded treatment. The systematic review included 23 various studies, 10 of which were randomized trials. The results across these studies showed a significant improvement in patients across all platforms.

Meditation continued to snowball through the decades and the likes of Joseph Goldstein, Jack Kornfield, and Sharon Salzberg created the Insight Meditation Society (IMS) by 1975. The IMS played a huge role in welcoming non-philosophical meditation in the West and promoted the idea of using it in leisure as well.

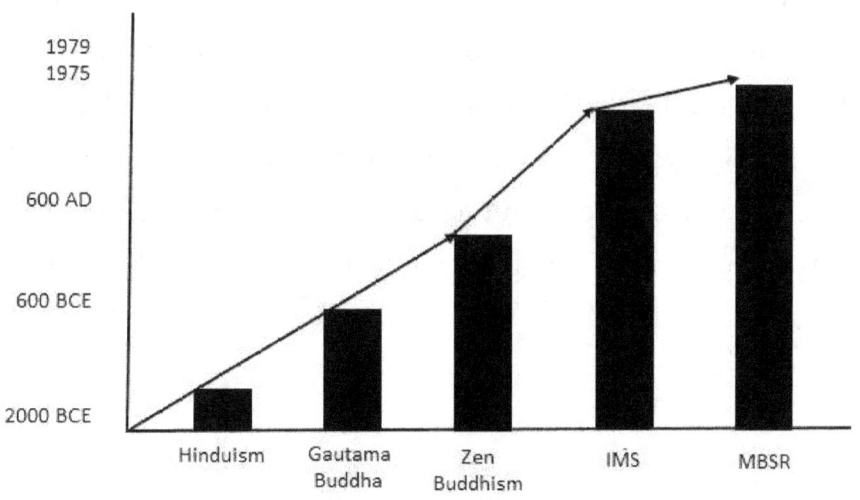

What Is Mindfulness?

I hope you enjoyed my history lesson and I'm sure your mind is curious as to what mindfulness is. The practice and perfection of mindfulness can come in many forms, including yoga and meditation. However, I'll focus on meditation because yoga may be out of your direct reach if you're obese and it's something you can consider at a later stage when that fat melts right off. Practicing meditation mindfulness can be enjoyed anywhere you choose, and you're welcome to listen to multiple video and audio tracks online or join a group session locally.

The definition of mindfulness roots in various areas of your life. The overall rule of this practice is to bring yourself to a precise moment in time and that moment is now. Your awareness of your direct environment becomes heightened and you focus on what you're doing. When you become accustomed to the practice, you'll overpower any feelings of your presence that would usually overwhelm you. So many people are unaware that they contain this skill from the day they're born but yes, it exists in you and practicing it will magnify it so you can access it anytime you need to. Isn't it great to know that you don't need to summon up a skill that has no roots in your mind? The roots are there, and I'll teach you to find them.

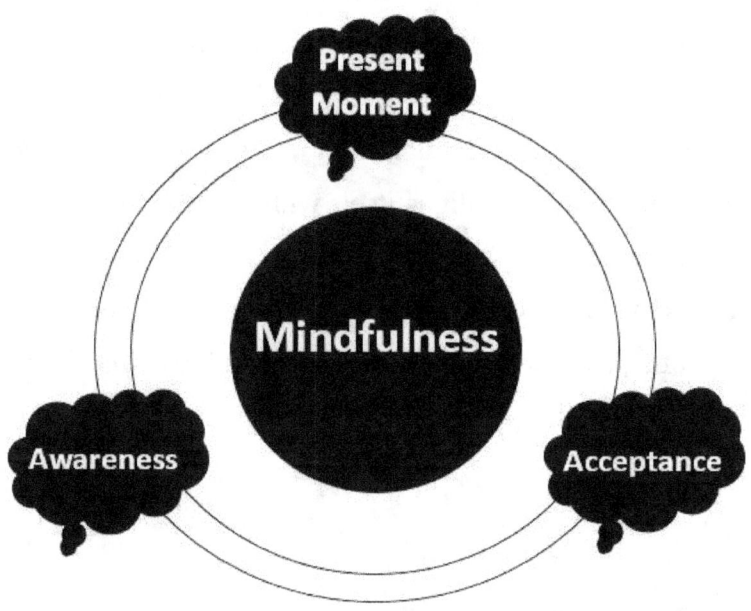

There's a valuable lesson to be learned in living in the present because you finally realize that you can't change the past or future, but your actions can cause a reaction. Being in the present is the only way you can cause a chain reaction to permeate throughout your future. So, what if you're overweight now? Nothing you do could ever take back all the times you did overeat but making a conscious decision to change that right now will change the future.

Mindfulness can also help you deal with your feelings because they take on a tangible form when you're able to connect with them in the present. Your thoughts, beliefs, and behaviors become real when you sit down and think them through thoroughly. When you learn to live in the here and now, life aligns itself with realistic ideas. Every time you feel the guilt about your previous choices, bring yourself back to a mindful state and accept the fact that you can't travel through time to alter your past choices. Welcome mindfulness into your life so that you can use the power of the present time to bring about the changes you need.

Using Ancient Practices to Reset Your Mind

Understanding the definition of mindfulness isn't the final stop. How does being present allow you to alter the future? It has nothing to do with science fiction or magic either. Mindfulness is a proven technique to change the circuitry in your brain because science tells us of another part of the brain which can't be seen physically but its existence has been used in psychotherapy for many years. Using this practice to change the way you think sources itself in medical science more than philosophy again. Franz Mesmer, who was a physician in Austria, opened himself to curiosity about mesmerizing people, also commonly referred to as animal magnetism.

Let's clear the air before you think you know where this is going. There's a massive difference between the hypnosis you see in Vegas and medical hypnosis. The latter has no "magic" or "tricks" involved. Typical myths about hypnosis involve people not remembering anything that took place and people having no control over their thoughts, feelings, and behaviors while under hypnosis. These are both total bullshit and fall under a separate category known as mentalism. Clinical hypnosis is the process of entering your physical and mental body into a deep stage of relaxation that resembles the delta stage of sleep. This is the stage your dreams enter your mind before you slip into the rapid eye movement (REM) dream stage.

However, in hypnosis, you don't sleep. Please understand this and don't assume you'll be under someone else's control and forget your journey. Hypnosis can be practiced at home as you do with meditation and the form I'll introduce you to is a combination of the two. You'll enter a relaxed phase and your subconscious mind, where dreams come from, will open to suggestion. Think about planting an idea in your brain and the only way the idea can latch on is by suggesting it to your subconscious mind. Any other level of consciousness will shrug the idea off. This isn't a theory and science supports the facts. This is the same concept that inspired the movie Inception in 2010.

This is one of the most powerful tools you can add to your arsenal when you're about to alter your overeating mind and shift compulsive or obsessive behavior for good. You are going to make use of self-hypnosis powerfully intertwined with mindful meditation. The only advice I can give you before I provide you with an exercise to follow is that this technique takes time to permanently plant your seed. Don't expect radical changes after one session because that's the most common mistake anyone makes. Your brain and consciousness are an intricate stellar map and this method should be practiced until the idea sticks with you. Even the movie tells you that it doesn't always take on the first try. You're going to nag your mind into submission.

My final word before we begin is that you should lie down because you might be someone who isn't physically comfortable sitting with your spinal column erect. Lie flat on a surface with comfortable clothes on while I guide you.

Meditative Exercise

I want you to focus on my voice, even if you're reading this. You can imagine my voice as any type of sound that's most attractive to you. My voice should sound clear in your mind and my words bring an odd sense of comfort to you. You're lying on your back and staring at the words in front of you. Can you feel how your body caresses the surface beneath you? Try and welcome the sensation against your skin because you notice there's a resistance in connecting with the surface below.

Listen to me and never remove your attention from my voice because every word will guide you into calmness. The gradual decline is happening slowly, but you can feel it. Take a deep breath through your nose and feel the air as it passes into your lungs. Count to three before you let it go and push it gently out of your mouth. Take another breath in and hold it before pushing it out slowly. Keep breathing like this and keep the breaths an even amount of time through the exhale and inhale. Feel how each breath raises your diaphragm slightly before it falls lower to the surface beneath you again.

Feel the thump of each beat as your heart finds its rhythm in your breathing. Your body is slowly releasing the resistance it held against the soft covers below your body. It feels like your body is melting into the surface and becoming slightly lighter with each breath. Continue breathing and looking at the words. Do you see any change in the words you're reading? They appear to be amalgamating with the white background as you continue. There's a soothing sensation that enters your physical body with every drop of air that passes through your vital organs; the same organs that felt heavy when you started. The pressure around your organs is lifting and your body keeps drifting further into the comfort of your bed.

My voice is caressing your soul and mind as you watch the words fraternizing with the background. They're growing bigger now but you don't question the size and gradual growth of them. There's a magnetizing rhythm that catches the attention of your retina. Follow the flow of these words and feel your heart rate slow down with more pressure exiting your body with the exhale of air. Your entire physical body is losing all the weight that held it in this consciousness. My voice travels through your mind as you realize the words are larger than ever. There's an undeniable comfort in the rise and fall of your body with every breath as you continue. You've never felt so calm before and you welcome it to take over. You can't move your visual focus from the words spinning around in front of your eyes. It doesn't matter how they move; you continue to follow the words in order.

You can feel your body submitting to the gentle surface below and the weight has lifted from your physical presence. Your heart is beating at a slower pace than you've ever noticed it before. You can't help but count the beats as you make sense of the gradual process of the words overwhelming you. Breathe in and out while you count each heartbeat. As you reach number 10, something new has happened. You're completely aware of the darkness that surrounds you as the words have consumed you. Your vision has opposed the scene you saw in the light and now you see a new image while your mind follows the words on their own.

There's an attractive light which beckons you closer, and for the first time, your mind has split into two visions. You can't feel your body anymore, but you can feel a presence in the form of moving closer to the light. It taunts you to come closer and there's an overwhelming peace in the light. All the fears you felt before this is fading away as you draw nearer to the light. You can see a silhouette of someone in the light, but you need to move closer. Keep breathing in through your nose and out through your mouth. Continue this slow and even flow of air through your body as your heart yearns to be closer to the light.

Follow your heart's irresistible guidance as you enter the visual distance from the light. The silhouette that lies in it resembles yourself. You can't see your face, but you know who this is. You have strong knowledge and acceptance of your subconscious mind that's kneeling on the ground. Listen to my voice and your heart's rhythm as you move even closer. The silhouette is becoming clearer and something is disturbing about it. Are they bound by chains? Your beats continue and you count three heartbeats before you arrive at the image of yourself. This indescribable calm that has possessed you suddenly shifts to worry as you realize the bondage that holds your subconscious mind prisoner.

The chains that bind them are not made of any substance that seems normal. You continue breathing and listening to my voice as you bend over and take a closer look at these chains. They remind you of a substance that resembles blubber. Are these chains made of blubber or fat? How is the bondage so strong if this is true? Your mind is curious, and you keep investigating the blubbering bondage. You can't touch it because it's only a mental image. You try aimlessly to feel the binding vines of fat that surround your image to no avail. You can feel the substance as your hand passes through, but you can't manipulate the image in any way.

You step back for a moment and gaze at this image. Your curiosity is fading and there's a new emotion taking its place. This is one emotion you're all too familiar with and its common name is sorrow. You're saddened by the image in front of you because this image is trapped in the bondage of self-creation. You notice your heart skip a beat and fear looms in your stomach. Take a moment and concentrate on your breathing as you acknowledge the deep sadness you feel. Don't shove the feeling away. Inhale slowly through your nose and hold it before you press it gently out of your mouth. Each breath of air brings a cooling sensation to your heart which has overheated from the image in front of you. Listen to your heartbeat as it finds an even rhythm again and allow the sadness back into your heart.

The image creates a knob in your throat, and you can feel a warm sensation touch your cheek as a tear escapes your eye. Don't be afraid and allow yourself to cry for this image. The warm wetness that caresses your cheeks soothes you. Your tears feel like heaven on your skin because crying is medicine for the soul. Allow your emotions to flow out through your physical eyes as you fear for the wellbeing of this image. Every tear that escapes brings you back to a deeper calmness and your cry turns into a forceful flow of emotion through your eyes.

As the tears dry up, you can feel the overwhelming sadness fade away. There's a new emotion creeping up on you and you fear the arrival of this one. It's another familiar emotion and the warmth enters through your toes first and travels slowly up your legs. The temperature is increasing in your lower belly before it reaches your upper torso and spreads down your arms.

Keep breathing as you notice an increase in your heart rhythm again. Your breathing remains even but your heart is beating faster with every breath. The warmth spreads further into your mind and finally, you place a name to this new sensation. The temperature is rising further while you recognize this immense feeling that has plagued you on so many occasions. This angry emotion pumps blood through your heart at a speedy rhythm now and the heat is overbearing.

You look over at the image bound before you and notice the crease in your brow as your anger rises. Rage is consuming your thoughts and feelings now because you're aware that you've done this. You take full responsibility for your actions and the image in front of you doesn't break for a moment. You continue breathing as you feel another sensation in your throat. Allow the sensation to overpower any resistance again. Suddenly, you feel this sound escape your throat as you scream because you've never felt angrier and more hurt before. Flow with the sound as it vibrates through every part of your being. You can feel the heat escaping with the sound waves that leave your throat.

The temperature gradually decreases in your body again and the new warmth is welcoming. You feel your heart slowing down but there's a new vigor in its rhythm. Every obvious thump pumps a new overpowering sense of compassion through every vein in your body. You feel sorry for the image in front of you and nothing is stopping you from breaking these bonds anymore. Your mind reaches a new level of understanding and you know what to do. These blubber chains cannot be broken from where you stand. You need to reverse yourself and return to the physical realm of being before you can break these chains.

Suddenly, you make yourself a promise while you stand over this image. "I promise that I will apply the changes needed to free you from this reality." As the words escape your mouth, the image finally raises their head. You find yourself staring at your own eyes and there's a strong magnetic pull back to the physical presence. Your heart gains a new, faster rhythm again and your physical body starts feeling the pressure of weight again.

The final glance from your image confirms the acceptance of your promise and you feel an overwhelming sense of trust in your promise. The image begins fading rapidly as you follow the sound of my voice and the harmonious drumming of your heart. You can feel the material of the covers under your skin again and the image has become nothing more than a distant light again. I want you to keep breathing evenly as you count slowly to ten. On the count of 10, you'll have the power to realign your vision as singular again.

The words are no longer part of you and you're no longer part of the words in front of you. You're surrounded by a deep sense of accomplishment, understanding, and faith in yourself as you take a moment to realign your visual presence in the here and now. Give yourself a moment to collect yourself before you continue to the next chapter and please listen to a few meditative sessions on YouTube and Audible.

Chapter 6: Let's Get Physical

Your body is your temple as your parents taught you, as well as your teachers in school, your spiritual leader, and even the internet. It's physically possible for you to retain your physique without having to climb mountains. The shift in overall health will permeate through your body and mind. Allow me to introduce physical movements using advice for obese people in mind.

Love and Respect Your Temple

There are so many physical changes that have taken place in your body since you began overeating. Gaining weight is only one of these changes. You've learned to repair your mind and your emotions, but your body is what carries the two. Your body goes through changes whether you're living it up like a health nut or you're sliding into the blubber stage.

Have you ever watched the 2007 comedy *Norbit*? Eddie Murphy is stuck with this enormous wife who isn't very kind to him on any level. After watching the movie, I struggled to get one scene out of my mind. The scene where Norbit's wife decides to go down the vertically challenged slide stunned me. Even though this shot is hilarious, to say the least, it's deeply disturbing. It was one of the many visuals that stuck in my mind and cumulatively made me change my future before I looked like her.

You need to find the happy medium of loving your body just as you do with your mind and emotions. You should respect your body by all means and take care of it as much as you can without obsessing over it either. I hated photos when my BMI placed me well into the obese range. I would find every excuse under the sun to avoid being in someone's shot because, quite frankly, I understand today that this is our way of avoiding the truth. I knew exactly how large I was, and I first thought it was best not to see these photos. However, that changed one day when I was unable to avoid a shot.

It was Christmas morning and the entire family was around when someone was clever enough to take a video without me noticing. They weren't trying to deceive me on purpose, but this person was going to England and they wanted a memory to take along.

It wasn't until a few weeks had passed before I saw this video and took a screenshot of one slide. Honestly, this was the end of the road for me. I've accumulated all these tics in my brain, images, and memories that nudged me in the right direction, but this one drove me off the cliff. We all have a breaking point and this one was mine. I always believed my uncle Bob was morbidly obese and found myself shamefully making it common knowledge. The video happened to capture us in one screen where I was sitting next to him and the truth was undeniable; I was just as large as my uncle Bob.

I'll admit, this didn't only send me over the edge, but it also hurt me deeply. I began questioning the loyalty of friends and family because not one person was honest enough with me. Why couldn't they tell me that I was as fat as my uncle every time I made fun of him? My emotions were bouncing off the walls and I was balling my eyes out for days while I stood in front of the mirror and taunted myself. I lifted my stomach flab and watched the jingle as it dropped back down. I wiggled my underarms and noticed the profound roundness of my buttocks. I spiraled into a deep depression and wouldn't allow anyone in. I was angry at family and friends. Why the hell did no one tell me I look like a baby hippopotamus when I wore my bathing suit to the pool? Did these people not care about me?

It took me two months to snap out of my rage and depression before I finally put my foot down. Enough was enough! That was my turning point and the reason I'm sharing this with you is that the kindest thing a loved one can do is be honest with you. Yes, it hurts to hear the truth and you may not agree for a long time, but the truth will set you free. Before you go any further into this guide, I want you to stand in front of the mirror and take a good look at yourself. While you're at it, take a few photos to keep for reference. I still have my photos today, and let me tell you something, they keep me in line.

There are multiple ways to love your temple and exercise is only one of them. Your body is a living, breathing organism and you need to treat it as such. Make sure that you fuel your body with the right fillers. It's not just what you eat and drink, but the programs you watch, the books you read, and even the radio channel you listen to matters. You're feeding your brain and soul and your body is perfectly in sync with them.

I want you to start listening to your body as though it's talking to you every day. Your body knows when you're full, dehydrated, hungry, craving something the body needs, and just bored. Focus on listening intently and with time and practice, you'll learn to hear what it's saying. Your body will also tell you when it's time to sleep. You need six to nine hours of restorative sleep every night. Remove any distractions that keep you awake and switch that damn television off at night.

Stop treating your body like a fragile piece of glass. You'll be surprised at what your body is capable of. It's not going to shatter into a million pieces when you begin moving it. You can't get anywhere on this journey without getting your blood pumping. It will be hard at first but if you keep listening to your body, you'll know what your limits are. Reducing your weight is only one tiny part of what needs to be accomplished. It's possible that your body has been strained for years and strengthening your core is essential. Your bones are the structure that keeps your weight, organs, skin, and muscles together. Some lightweight training will boost the strength of your bones with time.

Keep your body hydrated with water and health teas. Your recuperation journey won't become any easier if you're drinking excessive amounts of carbonated drinks and coffee that contain caffeine and sugar. Remember to stretch your muscles before any exertion because it doesn't only provide you with muscles less prone to injury, it also soothes the mind. Stretching is a common technique in yoga because it strengthens the mind, body, and soul.

Your brain becomes more susceptible to deterioration as you age and giving it some brain food will halt the process. You can teach your brain new skills by remaining curious. Haven't you ever wanted to learn a second language? Now's your chance to do that. Pick up new skills and challenge your brain with crosswords to keep the circulation flowing in your brain. You know exactly how much your brain plays a role in your current situation and allowing it to deteriorate won't make it any easier.

Your teeth, eyes, and ears are what connect you to the world around you. Keep your smile as gorgeous as the dentist can make it and use eye drops to keep your eyes in shape. Hell, buy yourself a pair of Ray-Bans if you want. Your ears are just as important, and you need to stop listening to the television loud enough to receive noise complaints from your neighbors every night. Keep regular appointments with all your physicians to check your teeth, eyes, and ears. Let's not forget to keep a close eye on any other potential health issues.

Also, you can become the next Gordon Ramsay. Allow your curiosity to drive your passion for cooking and experiment with various foods in this guide. Often, ingredients involved in any form of dieting can seem so boring but if you experiment with them, you'll surprise yourself. I don't want to brag but I've concocted some amazing dishes over the last few years, and fear not, I'll share a few with you. I want you to experiment with cooking and learn to love your body by expanding your experimentation. I'll provide you with the knowledge but it's up to you to use it as you see fit.

Finally, protect your skin from the sun and any other harmful contributors. I don't go out without spreading some sun protection factor (SPF) 50 sunscreen on and wearing a sun hat. I also use minimal make-up and purchase skin conditioners. Someone who suffers from obesity should seriously look after their skin because you want to become a slimmer person, and this won't go down well if you fail to care for your skin. I used bottles of cream with tissue oil to reduce as much of the stretch marks as I could. Your skin is about to go through massive changes, and you need to nurture it every step of the way.

Getting Physical When You're Obese

Now we get to the exciting part of moving your body physically. You may be wondering if it's possible to move your muscles without injuring yourself, but I assure you that I'll guide you to do just that. Registered Dietitian Peggy Pletcher says even sedentary obese people can ease into an exercise routine (Timmons & Pletcher, 2016). Intimidation is inevitable but you can overcome your fear if you gradually ease into a routine that's specifically created for obese people.

The American Heart Association recommends 30 minutes of moderate exercise five days a week for adults (American Heart Association, 2018). I know this is a frightening figure when you're obese. However, you're welcome to divide this into three 10-minute sessions in your workout days. 10-minute sessions will burn the same number of calories as one 30-minute workout. I began with a five-minute session six times a day for the first few weeks. I used a treadmill that counted the calories I burned as I walked. I never set the speed high or even programmed an incline. I simply walked for five minutes at a time because I felt like I couldn't breathe at first.

Your body will tell you how much you're capable of in one session and you should listen to every word your body speaks. Remember that this isn't a sprint, but a marathon. It's important to apply the ritual of exercise gradually so that you can engrave a new habit in your routine. Another essential part of easing into it means that you must stretch before you exercise. This decreases any chance of injuring yourself. A simple warm-up exercise includes standing with your feet slightly apart and your hands placed on your hips. Keep your back straight and bend over to the left before you come back up. Now bend over to your right and repeat this stretch five times to loosen up your waist and hips. Your spine should remain erect at all times during warmups.

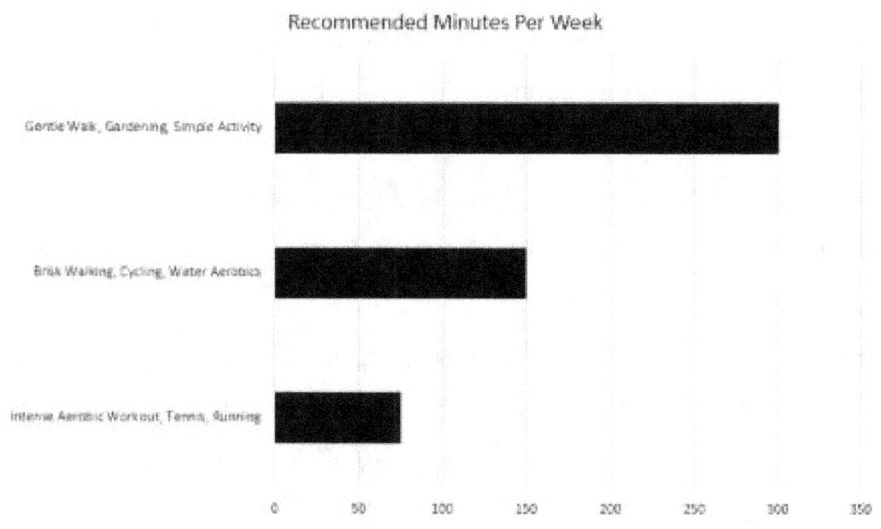

Now bring your feet together as you continue standing straight and bend one knee so that your foot faces backward and hold it for two seconds before releasing it. Do the same with both legs five times. Now you can bend over gently to reach as close to your toes as possible and raise your back straight again. Repeat this five times. Finally, you can stand straight and extend your arms upward in a flight position and hold them for two seconds before bringing them down again. Repeat this warm up five times. It's essential to warm all joints up before you do any exercise, even walking because your muscles aren't used to the strain of moving. Injuring yourself will deter you from exercising and that's not what we want. Stretches themselves shouldn't feel uncomfortable, and if you're feeling strain you should stop and change.

Another piece of advice I want to give you is that you should implement a breathing exercise daily too. This is similar to what you learned during your meditative session except you'll only be breathing. I used to find it helpful to do these breathing exercises for five to 10 minutes before my workout so that my heart is calmer. You take a deep breath through your nose and allow it to circulate in your lungs for two seconds before releasing it through your mouth. Continue doing this until you feel your heart rhythm slow to a healthier pace. You can do this exercise after you've completed your workout too.

I used headphones and listened to music while walking on my treadmill because you shouldn't watch the clock. Don't turn exercise into a routine that you dread. Make a playlist of your favorite music and listen to the songs that will inspire you. Walking was my favorite to start but you can use any exercise that you enjoy. You can get a stationary bicycle, a home stepper, or, my favorite in summer, swimming. Swimming is a great aerobic and cardiovascular workout, and who doesn't love getting wet when the temperature feels like hell on Earth?

The beauty of swimming is that it's a full-body workout and it doesn't matter how you move, as long as you move in the water. Obviously, don't just walk from one side to the other. Try and swim from one side to the other without touching the ground. You can even doggy paddle if that makes you comfortable. To install a new habit in your life, you should repeat the routine at the same time daily, just as you go to bed and wake up at the same time. Remember, you're reprogramming your brain and that includes your exercise schedule.

The reason I chose walking was that I wanted to get out into the world as soon as I was able to breathe while moving. I'm an extrovert and wanted to be among other people. The day I noticed my breathing didn't sound like a birthing exercise anymore, I went out to the park. I still walk today, and I've even joined park runs, morning groups of walkers, and nature hikes on weekends.

Walking gave me the ability to love what I do because you see something new every day. The clouds never have the same formation and the sounds of birds are always singing some kind of harmonious melody. I love nature, and since I began this journey I've become an avid hiker. My last hike was 20 miles to a lighthouse and back. That reminds me, if you live near a beach, make that your daily stroll. Walking on beach sand is amazing as the water tickles your toes, but it's also one hell of a workout.

I would strongly suggest that you stick to these cardio workouts before you take the next step. Once you're comfortable in your routine, you can join a group class that practices yoga or action sports. I admit that my action sports only kicked in when I'd lost half of my weight already, but I wouldn't swap them for anything now. My fitness levels rose when I joined a kickboxing club. I had no intention of learning to kick ass, but I wanted to target both my physical and emotional wellbeing. Yes, yoga does that but so does beating the crap out of a bag. My classes are every Tuesday night and I don't do it competitively. My fellow members are well aware of why I spend an hour in the gym every week. Every moment that has angered me throughout the week gets its own imaginative face on my bag and I open fire. Some people think I'm nuts, but I feel a new sense of freedom from all my emotional baggage when I'm done. I keep a journal every day as part of my CBT taught skills, and when I arrive at the gym I release every inch of pent up rage on the boxing bag.

The final word of advice I can give you personally on beginning an exercise routine is that you find support in other people. It's so easy to fall out of line when no one's watching. I'm fully aware of the embarrassment and shameful feelings that accompany obesity and overeating, but I also know how much a support group has helped me stay on track. You can easily find one on Facebook or Instagram and you should search words such as "obese workout buddies" or "obese exercise motivators." It's a concept as old as time itself and even weight watchers use the same strategy.

If it wasn't for my fellow ladies who were on the same path as me, I would have strayed for sure. Try and find a group that's local because you want to be able to meet with them in person. There's nothing to feel ashamed of because you're on the road to recovery. Those days of secretive pain inside you and being alone are over now.

Pragmatic Knowledge

I want to share some additional tips with you besides measuring your BMI. You need a starting point in your weight but the pounds on the scale are not your only enemy. I noticed how easy it was to lose the first few pounds because, honestly, it was water retained by my body. The first few pounds you lose in the first week or two are water retention. You want to watch the fat burn off your body, don't you?

There's one practical way to measure the physical loss of weight and that's by measuring your inches. It's one thing to say you lost 10 pounds but it's another to say you lost 10 inches. Gravity isn't reliable on its own and you need to measure the volume of weight that falls off as you progress through this program.

Buy yourself a measuring tape that people use in dressmaking. Find one that covers the circumference of your midsection. There are numerous points where I want you to focus on measuring yourself and you're about to begin with a diet diary. The first measurements you take can be entered in day one and you'll be measuring yourself every week. Please do this when weighing yourself too. You should never weigh yourself more than once a week because it's easy to fluctuate from day to day. To prevent discouragement, I've learned that weighing and measuring weekly is best.

Start at the top and measure the circumference of the widest part of your arm. Take note of where the measuring tape lies because you need to measure at precisely the same point every week. I used to measure on Mondays. Next, you can move the tape to your breasts and measure over your nipples. This goes for men and women. The next measurement takes place around your waist, in line with your belly button or navel. From there, you're going to measure your hips, and this can be done by placing the tape at the top of your pelvic line, just above your pubic hairline.

Now you move further down to measure your buttocks by placing the tape over the roundest part of your bum. From this area, you'll measure each leg individually again by reading the circumference of your top thighs. Always use the widest part you can see. Moving further down, you can measure your knees and then the widest area of your calves. Mark each measurement in your diary with the region that's been measured. When you do the same next week, you can take the accumulative loss of inches between all regions and that gives you the inches lost in that week.

Something you may not be aware of is that nearly every person on Earth has an inch difference between the left side of their body and the right side. I thought I was the only weirdo who got an inch difference in my arms and legs, but low and behold, my entire group was experiencing the same thing. Our coach then informed us that this was perfectly normal. Anyway, you won't find a deeper motivation than the first time you see how many inches you've shed, and an overwhelming sense of pride will latch on to you.

Move Your Body: Immobility

Some obesity sufferers have restrictions with their movements, and I want to focus on that for a moment. This section targets people who are immobile and can be carried out in a chair or even on your bed. I'm going to give you a routine to follow and each movement must be repeated 10 times. Let's begin.

Stretch your arms out into a flight position again and bring them forward to clap in line with your heart. Keep them straight throughout your movements. Next, you can roll your upper torso from side to side, lifting each shoulder and placing weight on the opposite shoulder. You just want to get movement into your upper body by doing this. Next, I want you to rest your elbows on the surface of the bed or armrests and circulate your wrists gently. Now reverse your direction and do this 10 times again.

Now I want you to sway your hips from side to side as though you're dancing while flat against a surface. Your one shoulder will move higher than the other as you do this. Next, you can start rolling your ankles. First in one direction and then in the next. This will be followed by bending your knees. Move your knees apart before bringing them back together when you're lying down, and if you're sitting you want to raise each knee as much as you comfortably can 10 times. Finally, I want you to become Shaky Stevens or Elvis Presley. Yes, vibrate your body while you count to 20, slowly. Shake every area of your body and do it as vigorously as you can.

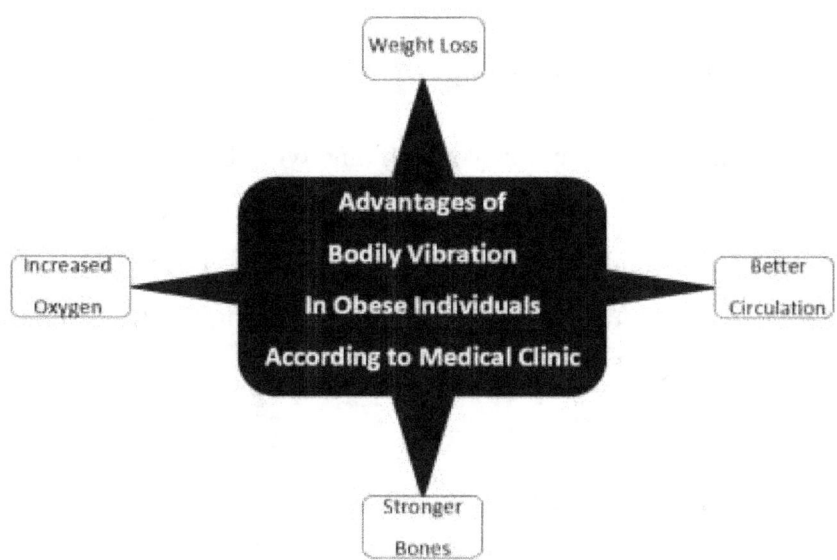

If you feel energetic after this workout, you can go another round. This exercise is solely for people who are completely immobile and should be followed closely by getting up and pursuing the aforementioned exercises.

Chapter 7: Set the Ball Rolling

You've learned to care for yourself and you know you're worth more than you believed last week. You'll find empowerment in new, reformed habits and you can finally set in motion the changes you deserve. Now we take the next step to changing your lifestyle by using proven techniques.

Empowering Health and Happiness

New beginnings are always frightening because there's uncertainty, fear of failure, and too many "what ifs." You're afraid to take the next step even though you know the devastating consequences of what's happened to you. Remember what I told you; it took me a few shoves before I realized enough was enough. The only way you can overcome fear is to face it head-on. I want to teach you more about CBT in this section and how practical exercises can help you overcome your fears.

What I want you to do is design a new "worksheet," if you can call it that. I'll include a diagram of the worksheet I want you to create but it will be simple. This technique will expose your true fears and all the emotional bondage that keeps you from getting back on the horse. This is not homework but rather a self-improvement strategy. Therapists refer to this as homework and, sure as hell, they give you a bucket load.

Give yourself five lines at the top. The only heading you need is "fears." In this section, you'll note all your fears as you perceive them, and it can include things such as:

- I'm morbidly obese and failure will make me gain more weight after the program.
- I'm afraid of giving up.
- I've tried so many diets before and they never work.
- My skin is going to hang like a half-mast flag; and
- People tell me that losing weight becomes difficult when I get older.

Now your second row of lines has the heading that reads "thoughts and emotions." How does each of your fears make you feel? Does the first one include thoughts of remembering past failures and feeling anxious? The second may be another recurring thought of giving up in the past, combined with fear and disappointment. The third is yet another memory lingering in your brain that tells you not to believe any advice you're given and doubt creeps into your mind. You don't feel confident in any program you're presented and feel depressed because there's no miracle cure. The fourth is thanks to reality television that has imprinted the image of people having loose skin after weight loss. There's a dread inside you and it depresses you further. The fifth fear is associated with other people and doesn't once say it's impossible. These five fears have only instilled a depressive and anxious mood in you.

The next part of your diagram can even be an obese stick man, depending on your drawing capabilities. Use different colored pencils to create blobs of representative circles in the areas for each fear. Blue can represent fear and red can indicate anger as an example. Go through your list of fears again and color circles in the region that you feel physically sick when a certain emotion or thought crosses your mind. Maybe you have an uncomfortable pressure in your chest when you feel anxious or you experience a light migraine when you become depressed.

Use your circles to color your little stick man, and finally place a percentage next to each color bubble. The pressure in your chest may be 75% threatening and the migraine may be 88% uncomfortable. Use a red pen for the percentages and write them neatly so that you can enter a new number under each one. While you're recording these color blotches, recognize the feeling in your body. Is your chest full of pressure right now? Accept that you can't physically change the pressure instantly and it will come and go. Allow it to be present in your body and acknowledge it but don't focus all your attention on it. In other words, don't obsess over the physical sensation you feel.

The final phase of this exercise is simple. You'll draw another five lines, and this will contain the heading "alternatives." Have a look at your list of fears once more and pause with each one. Is this fear realistic or does it root itself in your past experiences? Each fear should be questioned and undone until it's stripped naked. Here's a list of questions for each one:

- Do I have any evidence of my fear?

- Have I used the same approach with each one?
- What does research tell me?
- Have other people overcome this fear?
- Why do I fear this?
- Does other people's opinion of my choices matter?
- What matters most to me?

Delve into your rational thoughts and look at each fear from a third-person perspective. There's an undeniable truth in life; you can only face your fear by experiencing it. You can't do this by allowing your fears to control your decisions. Put this worksheet away now and you'll revisit it in two weeks again. You'll allocate new percentages to each color blotch on your sketch and read through it thoroughly again when you return to it. I can guarantee you that some of these fears are irrelevant upon revision because you've already noted a variance in your body.

If you see a change in percentages of a specific fear, it's time to enter your alternative. It may take time to enter each alternative because you're facing your fears before you record alternatives. Your third fear was entering a program that wouldn't work. Are you sure that this remains a fear after two weeks in the program? The word "alternative" means your alternative thoughts and emotions after facing your fear. You've seen a massive decline in your anxiety after losing 15 pounds and 10 inches over the last two weeks. Your alternative might be "this diet does work."

Keep this worksheet handy and keep referring back to it throughout your journey for inspiration because only you can plow through your fears. No one else can do it for you.

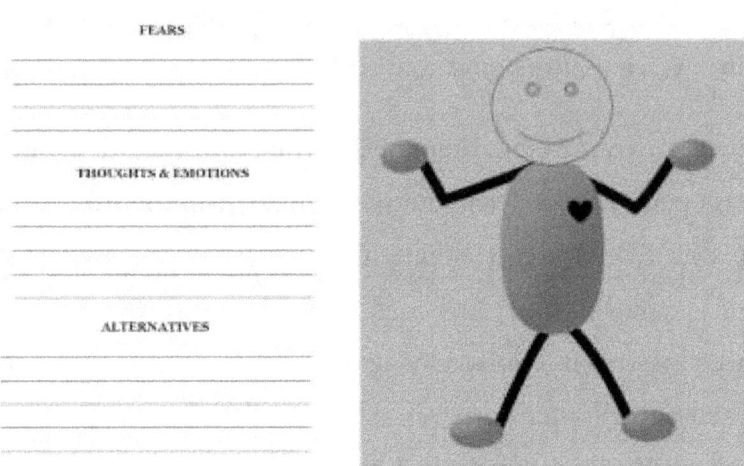

Breaking Bad: Establishing New Habits

Establishing new habits seems daunting at first, but alas, it isn't. I'll inspire you with another simple technique derived from CBT to install new software in your brain. Changing your habits are as simple as applying attention, focus, and repetition according to Psychologist Seth Gillihan (Gillihan & Hampton, n.d.).

The first part of habit alteration is to identify your habits. You did this previously and now you'll look at the list of habits you want to change. My list of habits included: eating at the speed of light, eating until I was about to pop, drinking fizzy sodas like water, procrastinating on the couch as soon as I got home, and eating one to five sweet treats a day. These are just some of my habits I've changed. Others included: being too lazy to bath before bed, watching Netflix until midnight, and snacking on popcorn or potato chips for the entire Netflix binge. I also had bad habits of not acknowledging my accomplishments and never treating myself to a reward when I achieved something. Basically, there's an endless list of possible habits you could add, and once you have your list we can move on.

Gillihan explains that insight isn't enough because even though people can identify the habits they'd like to change they often lack the action required to alter their negative thinking patterns. Making a change starts in your brain because it's the control center for your entire body. Habits can lie below your conscious level and they happen without you even noticing them. Your intentional actions derive from your limbic system. Your limbic system is in complete control of your automatic thoughts and drives the train to respond before you can give it a second thought. This is why you look at that donut and even though your logic is screaming for attention, it's overridden by your automatic thoughts and responses. This is why CBT directly targets your limbic system, and through repetitive behavior, it can replace these emotional thought cycles that prevent you from succeeding. The formal term for brainwashing your limbic system is called neuroplasticity.

You have set your goals and now it's time to make them as visible as possible. Remember to use reminders such as sticky notes. You should also place a target sheet on your refrigerator. Plan some new activities and begin with the easiest before you work your way to the most difficult. Start with the simplest task and set your alarm for the same time every morning. You're training your brain into a new rhythm and setting a precise sleep cycle will help you do that. Why not aim for waking ten minutes earlier tomorrow morning so that you can practice a meditative session or do your first five-minute exercise routine? Your energy is high in the morning and this is when you should take advantage of it. After doing your first entry in your schedule, take a moment to acknowledge the feelings you're experiencing. Focus intently on them. I want you to focus on every new entry for one minute before you move on.

Another repetitive habit I enforced in the morning was to eat my breakfast on the deck where the neighbors were in view. I know this sounds cruel, but it worked for me. This is how I overcame the speedy eating habits because I was aware of someone watching me. Every bite I took had to be chewed 10 times. I counted in my mind and wasn't allowed to swallow until I reached 10. Eating slower gives your brain a chance to catch up and release the chemicals needed to feel full. When I packed my lunch for work, I would read my list of allowed foods every morning, no matter how much I knew what it said. I'd also arranged with a colleague to eat lunch together every day so that someone was watching what I eat. I'd always remember to focus on the way I felt after each new alteration to my schedule so that I could realize the moments I didn't feel like throwing up from the excessive amounts I've eaten. Every change was recorded in my diary.

I would list activities in the afternoon that I enjoyed, one of which was my walk through the park. I would focus on the way the world looked different from yesterday and make mental notes on pleasurable encounters. I watched two birds feeding their baby while sitting on the bench after my walk. On Friday evenings, I would spoil myself and my family to a movie at the local theatre. I enjoy the theatre more than the cinema and we would visit one at least once a month. It was often dinner and a show, and my focus was intently on the on-stage show. This helped me consume my food slower and slower. Replacing my sugar drinks was difficult because I was addicted to them. I didn't start drinking water right away. I made myself cordial for the first few weeks and gradually made it weaker. Eventually, I was drinking water.

There isn't a doubt that you will deviate from your new routine and dive into old habits from time to time. When this happens, don't shoot yourself. Focus on the way your old habit made you feel and forgive yourself. The bottom line is that you need to replace your habits slowly and don't expect a complicated system such as your brain to change overnight. It will take time, and the more you repeat your new desired actions, the more they'll embed themselves in your automatic processes.

Down with the Cravings

Food cravings create a forceful desire inside you to eat or drink a specific product. As humans, we're prone to cravings from time to time, but you need to learn to recognize cravings that your body needs and cravings stemming from your past habits. Before I go in-depth here, I want to share a short story with you.

I was addicted to salty foods and I even asked the lady at the cinema to fill my extra-large popcorn only two thirds. The reason for this was because I needed to add a crazy amount of salt to my popcorn and if there wasn't space to shake the popcorn, the bottom bits would be tasteless. I craved the taste of salt and vinegar especially and this related to a craving.

As I taught myself to replace this habit over time, I found a natural spice called Pink Himalayan Salt. It's still salt, but a natural, unprocessed form of salt. I specifically bought the grinder with crystals inside. The same went for my pepper. I wouldn't use fine salt or pepper anymore and also replaced my vinegar with balsamic vinegar. I'm not going to lie when I say it tasted awful for the first few weeks. However, once I grew accustomed to the new taste, I loved it. I can't stand the taste of regular salt anymore, and since I made this change I stopped craving heavy doses of spices over my food. Sometimes we crave something our body needs but we use the wrong product to entice the cravings.

Cravings result from brain activity related to your habits. You may crave something unusual and you can't understand why in some cases. You could be craving something you're familiar with on the other hand. This can mean that your body requires something deficient and there are simple replacements for each.

There could be a lack of magnesium in your system if you're craving chocolate. Chocolate isn't the only source of magnesium. You can counter this craving with spinach, avocado, or almonds. When your body is screaming for sweet products, you are shy of chromium, carbon, phosphorus, sulfur, and tryptophan. Garlic and broccoli contain chromium. Raw or whole dairy products contain carbon. Wild tuna, organic beef, and soaked sunflower seeds contain phosphorus. Garlic and onions can fill your sulfur needs, and finally, organic eggs or chicken and fresh seafood can give you tryptophan.

Your craving for bread means you need nitrogen, and this is contained in organic meat, spinach, and wild seafood. You need calcium when you crave for excessively fatty or greasy foods. This can be replaced with sardines, cultured yogurt, and raw milk or cheese. Cravings for tea and coffee indicate that you require phosphorus, sulfur, sea salt, and iron. Sea salt can be found in Celtic sea salt or Himalayan salt crystals and iron is contained in organic beef, soaked lentils, and liver. Carbohydrate cravings include a desire for biscuits, rice, pasta, and potato chips. This indicates a shortage of magnesium or chromium again. It can also indicate a hormonal or adrenal imbalance in your system, and you can counter this with a bath. Add a cup of Epsom salts to your bath at night and soak for 20 minutes to replenish this need.

Cravings for alcohol means you're deficient in potassium, calcium, avenin, glutamine, and protein. Potassium comes from bananas, wild salmon, organic beef, broccoli, and avocado. Avenin can be replaced with soaked barley or oats when you're desperate. Glutamine can be fixed with cottage cheese, unpasteurized dairy, asparagus, and wild fish. Protein is found in organic meat, chicken, wild fish, beans, and lentils. Craving for a soda can indicate a need for calcium found in dairy. Chloride means Celtic sea salt and adrenal support foods include root vegetables, apples, beets, and berries.

Acidic food cravings mean you lack magnesium again. For the ladies, when you suffer from cravings during your premenstrual period, you are short of zinc. This can be replenished through eating chickpeas, cashews, or organic beef. Craving cheese in any form would indicate a need for essential fatty acids. This can include ghee, olive oil, coconut oil, and genuine butter. Stay away from margarine filled with trans fatty acids! Craving red meat or ice means you lack iron. Finally, craving fish indicates a shortage of iodine. Iodine can be found in saltwater vegetables like seaweed, wild seafood, raw cheese, and organic eggs.

Cravings can be a tempting magnet of transgression on your path, but they could also indicate a desperate shortage of vital vitamins, minerals, and chemicals required in your body. That's why it's important to handle them correctly. However, if you notice cravings that linger endlessly and don't subside by replenishing these minerals, you can stop them dead in their tracks with simple advice.

Drink a glass of water every time you feel a slight urge to eat something. You can include a glass before every mealtime too so that your body doesn't confuse thirst with hunger. Keep a significant protein intake in your diet to suppress the cravings you suffer from. The Department of Nutrition and Exercise Physiology, University of Missouri, Columbia concluded that obese men managed to reduce their cravings by 60% during weight loss programs when they increased their protein intake by 25% (Leidy et al., 2011).

Use your distraction skills to create a distance between yourself and the craving. If you feel yourself instinctively wanting a bar of chocolate, bring your thoughts to something else swiftly. A busy mind keeps away idle thoughts. Another tip is to plan your meals, and we'll get into this soon enough. This serves two purposes though because you have something to look forward to when you plan well, and you prevent yourself from getting too hungry at once because this leads to cravings. Cravings are also activated by emotional distress and when you keep your stress levels below par, you can curb these nasty hindrances.

Spinach extract is a new product on the market and can be useful in curbing a few cravings if you look at the list above. One teaspoon of the extract can remove your urge to eat chocolate and sugary treats. Once you dive into the details of your new diet; you'll also prevent cravings from creeping up on you. Even sleep deprivation can mimic the intense urge you feel for a certain product. Make sure you're getting enough sleep to prevent this.

The greatest piece of advice I can share with you is so practical that you'll kick yourself. Remove the products you crave from your home, office, car, and anywhere you frequent. I have a new habit when shopping for groceries or even just a few top-ups throughout the month. I make sure I shop on a full belly. The moment you walk down the aisle with temptation, and you hear the grumble in your stomach, you're bound to buy all the things you shouldn't. Don't ever shop on an empty stomach.

Chapter 8: Preparation for Alteration

The internet is filled with stories of miraculous magnitudes. You need to identify fact from fiction before you follow concrete advice on secrets that aren't so clandestine. There's a simple emotional direction you should steer away from and use expert advice to shift direction to the right emotions. The mental preparation you're looking for is more pragmatic than you could imagine.

Low Carb Diets: Myth or Fact?

We're finally easing into the part that's going to change your life. Before we jump ahead into the diet involved, we'll have a look at some myths and facts.

Do low carb diets make me eat huge amounts of protein?

I feel that this can count as a rhetorical question because I've already proven the benefits of a higher protein diet by providing a scientific study. Moderate intake of proteins is essential besides curbing your cravings. Low carb diets focus on a happy medium intake of protein and feed your body with essential amino acids. However, meat products shouldn't be highly processed; therefore, organic or organ meat is preferred.

Is there enough variety in these diets?

This is a *low* carb diet and not a *zero*-carb diet. You replace an excessive amount of carbohydrates with protein, moderate fruit intake, vegetables, healthy fats, seeds, nuts, and certain dairy products. You're still eating every food group and only changing specific ingredients. I found countless recipes and my experimentation in the kitchen went through the roof because there isn't a food group missing. Don't fall for people's self-soothing concoction of excuses.

There are so many restrictions on this diet

Another lie told by people who don't realize that anyone who cuts out processed food is already on a low carb diet. Unfortunately, the market is being flooded by endless new products and lazy foods which have been processed so many times that the product doesn't even taste real anymore. I call processed food plastic, and if you lose the taste for plastic, you'll find that nearly any recipe can be altered to include natural, organic food that tantalizes your taste buds.

How am I going to fulfill my energy needs if I don't eat enough carbs?

This is what you want happening in your body. Once your body has depleted the carbohydrates, it relies on burning fat for energy. Besides, fat doesn't act as a rollercoaster and leaves you crashing when the sugar rush wears off.

Isn't this just another fad that will pass with time?

Modern foods are filled with processed carbs and refined sugars. Why is low carb dieting considered a new "trend" when it's the oldest existing foundational diet? We ate natural products before this new age crap we eat today. Do these people spreading falseness honestly believe that cavemen ordered McDonald's when they felt hungry? Have they ever seen an enactment of a fat caveman? In ancient times, humans lived off the natural world and it's only in modern-day records that obesity exists on such a large scale.

I thought fat was a recipe for heart disease

Healthy fats reduce your triglycerides, raise healthy cholesterol, curb diabetes, and aid blood pressure. Triglycerides are one fine indicator of heart disease. It's high amounts of processed and refined carbohydrates, trans fatty acids, and saturated fat that increase all the risk factors according to the Heart and Stroke Foundation (Rosenbloom, n.d.).

I've heard that low carb diets deprive us of fiber

These myths get my panties in a bunch. You don't need bread to attain fiber because you're getting plenty from coconut oil, nuts, seeds, and all those delectable leafy green vegetables. You'll receive all the fiber you need without eating like a rabbit.

My brain needs glucose to function in the day

Oh, my word! I can't believe the myths I'm encountering online. So, these people believe that glucose is the only product that fuels your brain? I'm sorry but the people trying aimlessly to convince you of this need some brain fuel urgently because theirs are malfunctioning. Our brain needs glucose or ketones to repair itself, restore functions, keep acuity, and sharpen your attention like a pencil. Protein imitates glucose in your blood. This process is called gluconeogenesis, and non-carbohydrate carbon substrate proteins released in your bloodstream are converted into glucose or ketones for your brain. Protein is a glucogenic amino acid or no-carb precursor.

Is ketosis dangerous?

I've mentioned ketones, and your body uses protein to start burning fat once the glycogen stores run empty. This is what we call ketosis and healthy fatty acids are released into your bloodstream before they're turned into ketones and couriered up to your brain. To answer your question, no, ketosis is not dangerous. I know the name sounds very similar to ketoacidosis, but this is a completely different process. People who suffer from diabetes type one can experience a life-threatening number of ketones in their bloodstream that they're unable to control. Ketones are very much a controlled process in ketosis.

General Secrets to a Balanced Diet

I'm going to share the secrets and explain "state the obvious" guidelines of a low carb diet with you. You may know some of them and others will clarify some additional questions you might have. The basic principles of following a low carb diet include a few factors and they can be instituted in any order that serves you best.

The number one rule is that you should eat when you're hungry. This isn't some fasting game and you're causing a chemical reaction in your body that deprives you of energy when you starve yourself over a prolonged period.

Rule number two means you should learn to read the labels of everything. Become an investigator who purchases everything after you've read the label back to front. This doesn't only go for sauces, oils, peanut butter, yogurt, vanilla extract, marinades, spices, bouillon cubes, starch thickened sauces, and horseradish. It's just as important to read the label on non-edible products such as chewing gum, personal hygiene products, and medication. Shampoo, sugar scrubs, cough syrup, face masks, and even products containing honey can interfere with your blood glucose levels and halt weight loss.

Rule number three tells you to hide temptations. Make sure your kitchen and bedroom cabinets are free from all tempting carbs. This includes alcoholic beverages and crackers. Don't allow yourself to wake up in the middle of the night and be able to satisfy a random carb craving. Refer back to the cravings section and you'll find something wholesome to replace each craving with.

Rule number four tells you to expect a transitional phase. Your body is going from using carbs for energy to burning fat. Of course, you'll experience a transition in your energy levels. Don't stress because this won't last long. Just hang in there.

Rule number five is never skipping a meal. I know this is a factor in many diets but in low carbs diets, it's very important. Make sure that you eat three wholesome meals a day and have carb friendly snacks in-between to keep your body fueled throughout the day. Low carb dieting is not fasting and sending your blood glucose levels dangerously low won't help the hormonal processes that need to take place.

Rule number six explains that you should be careful of any "low carb" products. Bread, protein bars, pasta, ice creams, and even tortillas come in a so-called low carb variety. Beware of these products because the ice creams contain sugar replacements that end in the letters 'ol,' such as sorbitol. These are no good for you and you should make stevia your default sugar replacement. Low carb starch products and pasta, for example, will slow your weight loss and should be used sparingly, if at all. Low glycemic index (GI) bread products still contain sugar. The only difference is that it releases the sugar slowly into your system. The reason we maintain a minimal intake of fruit is because the fruit is rich in fructose. Even though this is natural sugar, it's still sugar.

Rule number seven tells you to focus on the right foods. Remove any processed, refined, and heavily packaged foods. Start shopping for wholesome organic products that are farm bred and not mechanically engineered, hormone-induced growth products. Eat loads of healthy fats and those include avocado, nuts, almonds, chia seeds, coconut, fatty fish, dairy, and eggs. Your metabolism can be boosted naturally by eating loads of chilies because it increases your body's temperature. Add jalapenos and homemade salsa to your daily diet. Stop fearing all fatty foods because your grandmother told you to. It's an automatic response we have and "fat equals weight gain" becomes a core belief. You're forgetting the process of ketosis, which is burning fat and you need the fat in your diet to avoid carbohydrates.

Rule number eight includes finding a balance between food and your physical prowess. Your daily routine should include 20% physical activity and 80% consumption of healthy foods.

Rule number nine tells you to replace your carbohydrate shortage with healthy fats. This means that you aren't allowed to skimp on anything other than carbs themselves. Your maximum carb intake daily shouldn't exceed 25 grams. Keep listening to your body. I cannot emphasize this enough, and your body will tell you how many carbs you need. A certain amount of carbs may work for one person and not the next. Use your gut instinct to tell whether your headaches, mood swings, sleep disruption, and energy levels are ultimately too low. Monitor your carb intake closely so that you can adjust any modifications necessary.

Rule number ten tells you to follow the correct order of importance for maximum benefit. The correct order is fat, protein, and carbs. Your daily intake should contain high fat, moderate protein, low carbohydrate intake to succeed. You can multiply your body weight by one and a half to attain your average protein intake in ounces daily.

Rule number eleven explains that you should make sure your expectations are realistic and don't expect to lose weight overnight. I know the internet and reality television is filled with miraculous stories, but you'll only set yourself up for heartbreak. Rome wasn't built in a day, right? You certainly didn't gain the weight overnight and you can't expect to lose it that way either.

Rule number twelve tells you to prepare for on the go rushes. Make sure your refrigerator is stocked with ready to go meals because a hungry lion can ravage it when there's nothing else available. Keep supplies of shredded chicken, cheese, boiled eggs, and steamed broccoli. Have an abundance of snacks to keep you from reaching the boiling point of hunger. When you suffer from the midnight snack attack, there's a solution to that too. I have a simple trick to combat these midnight munchies and that's a thickly sliced portion of cucumber with either cheese or butter on it. I eat this and follow it with a glass of warm water. Plan your weekly lunches too. This is essential if you work because no one can foresee the future and you don't know what the day will bring. You certainly don't want to arrive home with the appetite of The Village People.

Rule number thirteen tells you to avoid constipation when you're on a low carb diet and that's by keeping yourself hydrated with two glasses of water when you wake up and another six strategically placed throughout the day. Besides, the only combatant for water retention is water. When your body stores excessive amounts of water it's due to there being a lack thereof.

Rule number fourteen reminds you to keep your nutrient intake dense because your body needs 50 essential nutrients a day to balance physiologically. If you keep track of your numbers and the nutrients in each item on your recipe list for the day, you should get an estimated value of your intake.

These are some of the "laws" I live by and until today, I haven't changed them. Dieting is not a temporary solution and you need to change your life permanently to impact future success too. I've added a few more tips to get you excited. These are not rules but they certainly can make the transition easier for you.

Tip number one: Use veggie juice to curb cravings in the beginning. You can use any of the low carb vegetables to create a four-ounce juice in a blender that you drink after your meal. Starting a low carb diet is challenging and this can help you get through the first week.

Tip number two: Replace your cracker snackers with hard cheese. This is simply because low carb diets often make us feel like we have nothing to spread cheese on. But wait, you can spread soft cheese on hard slices of cheese. You have to admit that this sounds enticing.

Tip number three: Use romaine lettuce to create "hamburger buns" and enjoy the likes of beef burgers, tuna burgers, and chicken burgers. You can do the same with wraps. Lettuce provides a crunchy experience when turned into a wrap and the taste is out of this world when you use the right fillings.

Tip number four: Don't allow your vegetables to be boring. You can stuff veggies with protein and turn it into something you see on the cooking channel. Think about beef stuffed green bell peppers.

Tip number five: Leafy green vegetables contain slow absorbing carbohydrates and the good news is that the butter and olive oil you smother them in are further preventing the absorption of carbs.

Tip number six: Cauliflower is the gateway product to replace many unhealthy options. You can create a pizza crust, rice, mash, and even muffins with cauliflower. It's a versatile vegetable that offers all the benefits you require, and the only setback is the gas. Yes, you read that correctly. Cauliflower is amazing and can be used for and on anything. However, it does give you excess gas.

Tip number seven: Squash is another miraculous vegetable and you can create delicious spaghetti from squash. Zucchini or marrow can also be shaved and turned into a pasta alternative.

Tip number eight: Finely minced apple can be added to a quarter cup of water. This acts as a great substitution for flour. This means you can bake brownies without flour.

Tip number nine: Now this is the golden secret I wish to provide you with. *You can still eat chocolate* in moderation, but you should stay away from all the shop bought chocolates, even the darkest kind. You can make your own chocolate at home with a few ingredients. Take four tablespoons of unsweetened cocoa powder, a quarter cup of thick coconut milk, one teaspoon of liquid stevia, one tablespoon peanut oil, and a quarter cup of fine coconut. Stir the cocoa powder and milk together for two minutes before you gradually add the oil. Now you add stevia, fine coconut, and a drop of sugar-free vanilla extract. Freeze your chocolate for two hours and voila, you have carb-free chocolate. This is the best "secret" to a low carb diet in my opinion.

The Big Emotional Numbers to Remember

I know everyone will experience differences in their journey. However, I can guarantee you that certain foods will make you feel a certain way and that's one topic no one talks about. I experienced a vast fluctuation of emotions through my journey and they do taper down eventually, but until they do, you need to know that they exist. Low carb diets, fortunately, provide you with many soul-soothing ingredients and I'll share a few with you. I've discussed the chemicals and hormones with you earlier, but now I want to enlighten you on their potential benefits and the foods that provide these chemicals to you on a silver platter.

Dopamine is the motivational hormone in your body, but it does wonders for you. Hospitals use dopamine to treat patients who go into shock that's been caused by trauma, heart dysfunction, and a few other medical emergencies. Why do you think they do this? Dopamine urges you to seek pleasure and this is how it can alter your mood when you're feeling low. Products that contain dopamine are eggs, poultry, seafood, and various proteins.

Vitamin D is another player in the field and regulates your calcium and phosphorus. Besides this, it's known to elevate your mood. Have you ever stepped into the fresh air outside while the sun dances off your skin? You gain vitamin D naturally from the sun and even children experience a mood shift. Egg yolks and milk are great sources of vitamin D.

Vitamin B12 is the next on my list. Both vitamin B12 and folate are used to decrease depression. Ingredients that contain both are broccoli, lentils, and dark leafy greens. The vitamin on its own can be found in cottage cheese and salmon.

Fiber plays its own tune, besides keeping you regular. It contains sugar inhibiting molecules that slow down the absorption of sugar and increase your levels of serotonin. Serotonin is a "feel good" natural remedy. Serotonin can be found in beans, peas, and Brussels sprouts.

I want you to realize something once and for all: dieting isn't only used to lose weight. You've entered this journey to become a healthier individual and that includes your mental, physical, emotional, and mindful state. Allow the food you consume to direct the flow of your emotions and avoid foods that make you feel grossly emotional.

Preparing Yourself Mentally

You've been armed with all the information you need but now the time has come to put the information into action. Do you feel ready for this? I know you've spent time in practices that prepared you mentally, but I want to give you a few more pointers.

All the data you've been recording and the goals you've set need to come together now. Bring all the data in one book to keep track of your journey easier. Think of this as your plan of action. No person can enter a strategic mission without their plan of action. This extends to sports, business, and even psychology.

Have you watched sports movies? There's so many of them, and if you watch one, you'll notice how they sit in the locker room before the game and strategize their movements. Yes, there are times these strategies can be compromised in the heat of the moment, but a coach will never send their team in without a game plan. The best game plan and the teams that follow through with them is the reason why many games are won. That's why football teams pay exorbitant fees for their coaches because the coach is the strategy man. The stronger his plans have proved through his career; the more people are prepared to pay for him.

Nevertheless, you're piecing the puzzle of your game plan together now. That's the only solid way to approach the field. Everything else you've learned has only given you supplementary assistance in your strategy, but now you'll finally put it together. Follow these steps to make a list of what your diary must contain.

1. List your goals. This includes your weight loss goals, your lifestyle changes, and future possibilities of new encounters.
2. Create a detailed meal plan and shopping list for your diet. Prepare yourself for at least a week in advance with this. The foods you should include will be shared soon.
3. Invest some time and energy into your workout routine. You can include a financial investment if you need someone to help keep you in line. Hire a personal trainer if you can. Otherwise, you can enlist your friend.
4. Keep a separate journal that will become your food log. You need this separate because you want to compare your diet and meal plan to what you ate.

5. Choose date entries for the timeline you want to reach your milestones with weight and inches lost. Highlight these entries to remind you to weigh and measure yourself.
6. Keep working on your self-esteem and refer back to the notes in this book to boost it every time it runs low. You can diarize a day each week where you should assess your emotional state again.
7. Rewards should be jotted down because you want to look forward to them. Make sure you use a pen so they can't be changed.
8. Keep entries of contact numbers for support from friends, family, and the support group you've pinpointed in your location.

WEEKLY PREP SCHEDULE	MONDAY	TUESDAY	WEDNESDAY	THURSDAY	FRIDAY	SATURDAY	SUNDAY
GOALS		X					
WEEKLY GROCERIES						X	
EXERCISE SCHEDULE	30 MIN	30 MIN		30 MIN	30 MIN	30 MIN	
FOOD LOG ENTRY	X	X	X	X	X	X	X
WEIGH AND MEASURE	X						
EMOTIONAL ASSESSMENT			X				
REWARD (IF EARNED)							X
CONNECT WITH SUPPORT GROUP		X			X		

Planning is the way you find the mental strength to jump into the dietary fire pit. Let's do this.

Chapter 9: Detoxifying Your Temple

Detoxing your body is essential before you alter the nutrition you consume permanently. Your body is toxic from the poor intake you've had until now. Your digestive system is in tatters and the need for an enhanced gut function is more now than ever. I'll share an overview of the various kinds of detoxification you can partake in before you jump in the deep end.

How Do Detox Diets Promote Healing?

The truth of the matter is that you've likely been binge eating for years now. This has created an entirely new "normal" in your eating lifestyle and your body. The definition of the word detox is a process or period in which you cleanse the body of toxins or poisons gradually by removing them one by one or all together.

My detox was a gradual weaning process. Imagine someone who's been addicted to cocaine and heroin. They spend weeks in detox before their bodies come to terms with the change. You cannot rip the band-aid off instantly; these toxins must be removed slowly. Your body has relied on them to function as it deemed it to be normal for a long time now.

Cocaine addicts suffer severe withdrawal symptoms when their narcotic addiction is swiftly removed from their system. Their body goes into a stage of shock and craves the so-called norm it's used to, sending a shockwave of urges through every muscle in their body. You've learned about the physiology behind your hormones and the psychology behind your impulsive urge for the irresistible substance your body craves. Your body is like a child who's afraid of change. It doesn't know what comes next and it goes into a frantic panic when faced with foreign proposals.

Your biological body has grown accustomed to these toxins, no matter how disruptive they are, and if you think you can suddenly change from eating five boxes of chocolates to a large salad without detoxing, you're hopelessly wrong. Your body will enter a shocking withdrawal phase, and this will only help you slide back into your old habits to feed the irresistible urges that you once obsessed over. Almost every diet on the market suggests that you enter a detox before you play ball with the diet itself. This allows your body to ease into the changes about to take place.

If you don't enter a diet using some form of detox, your body will reject the changes, and mentally, physically, and emotionally you'll rely on your obsession and compulsive behavior to cope again. This is how detoxing promotes healing because you're changing a habit gradually to prevent relapse.

The Clockwork of Your Digestive System

I want to teach you about your gastrointestinal tract (GI) so that you can understand the process in your body. Doctor Emmanouil Karampahtsis from Phoenix explains that any major disturbance in your digestive system can have complex consequences (Karampahtis, 2016).

You've learned about the complex diagram that exists in your neurology and your endocrine system. Your digestive tract is connected to these systems. Your GI is a complicated network of organs that work harmoniously with each other. The main focus of this network is to help your body process foods that you consume. This includes organs and muscles that create a chewing movement, right down to the waste excretion from your body. Muscular contractions are what help you chew, swallow, and even stimulate movement to aid in the mixture of your food with digestive juices in your stomach.

Digestive juices vary from one organ to the other and they include bile, saliva, pancreatic fluids, and stomach acid. As your hypothalamus and endocrine system instruct the production of these digestive juices, your body attains vital nutrients from the foods processed in these organs by collecting it and sending it into your bloodstream. Your limbic system is in charge of the muscle contractions and juice production of each digestive organ. Your digestive tract also contains serotonin, dopamine, and nitric acid, similar to your nervous system. Your GI regulates more neurotransmitters than your brain.

Nevertheless, the nutrients absorbed in these digestive fluids are essential for the health of many organs in your body. They promote growth, energy, cell restoration, and more. Your GI tract is responsible for excreting the waste from your body, or in this case, the toxins.

Your throat secretes saliva that targets starches, fats, and carbohydrates, and the liver releases bile to combat fats. Your pancreatic fluids remove starch, protein, and fat. Your stomach deals with protein, and your small intestines set their eyes on starch, protein, and carbohydrates. Now, it's important to remember that carbohydrates are converted to glucose and I've taught you that protein can do the same through imitation of carbohydrates. Therefore, your small intestines can use protein to create glucose instead of carbohydrates. Our bodies get into a rhythm where each of these organs is accustomed to certain additives entering your body. If you make a sudden and drastic change in this flow, these organs will seek the nutrients they need elsewhere, which can leave you feeling ill.

This is why it's crucial to introduce a new rhythm to these organs in morbidly obese cases by tricking them. Your liver will maintain its regular processes because you're not removing fat from your diet. You're simply replacing it with a healthier fat that contains the nutrients your body needs. Your throat will continue to process protein as a glucose substitute and you're not depriving it for even a moment. Your pancreas and small intestines will continue as normal because they continue receiving mostly the regular substances they're used to. If you're comfortable enough, you can use a fasting technique to rest these organs before a new rhythm is introduced.

Achieving Improved Gut Function

Detoxing or cleansing your system offers a bright future for your gut health. I was surprised to learn that 70% of my immune system's cells reside within my gut. That alone explains why toxins can create bountiful problems in my overall health. Your stomach is the first line of defense against attacks from pathogens in your body. Pathogens are bacteria that cause disease and the defensive bacteria in your gut are supposed to eliminate the bad. If your gut is indisposed, you're automatically predisposed to obesity, among various illnesses. Other possible consequences of an ailing gut are impaired brain function, emotional instability, and a weakened immune system.

Detox programs don't only aid in weight loss and dieting, they have many other benefits associated with them. These include:
- Less diarrhea or constipation.

- Lowered levels of depression.
- Little to no fatigue.
- Improved allergies.
- Removal of mood swings.
- Reduced bloating.
- Reduced headaches.
- Freedom from joint pain.
- Reduced inflammation.
- Fewer skin problems.
- Removal of the chance of attention deficit.

A detox plan allows you to systematically replace foods that cause these issues with foods that promote gut health. Various programs enhance healing your gut and creating a sealant against alien invaders. The proper guidelines can help you attain probiotics in your stomach, which means that your defensive bacteria increases. Many detoxes also cleanse and reset your bowel functions by encouraging fiber-rich foods. Someone who's suffered obesity and poor gut health for a long time can also be resistant to insulin and suffer from organ inflammation that causes a delay in weight loss.

The diet I'll provide you with will ensure gut health by replenishing your storage of key nutrients and the detox guidelines will take you one step further. Let's delve into the details of detox options before you begin your new life.

The Various Options

I used a simple method of detox that allowed me to gently remove poisonous toxins from my system. I never entered a fasting stage or ripped away every pleasure known to man in one day. I'll share a few detox methods with you that can help you achieve the results you're looking for without frightening your system into retaliation. I will end this section with one form of fasting that I would approve of.

The number one rule I want to cover, though, is that you should avoid any detox plans that remove all toxins in one go over an extended time frame. These problematic plans include those that restrict your portions immediately. I've been obese and I know what it feels like to try and go from eating an overflowing mountain of food to one fist full of greens that you weigh on the kitchen scale. Don't chance the risk of slipping back into your old habits. Trust me on this one.

Three Day Plan

Let's begin with a rush detox or a three-day detox. I'm not going to even bother focusing on any shorter length of time because you can't possibly remove harmful toxins by the hour and expect the changes to embed themselves. You're welcome to downsize the portions you're used to for this detox plan to what makes you comfortable. However, I'm going to advise that you keep it under one dinner plate or breakfast bowl for each. The snacks are essential because they'll add extra fuel between meals.

The first day will include removing any additional refined sugars from your diet. This means that you're not even allowed to chew gum because your salivary glands will pick this up. Increase your water, green tea, and warm freshly squeezed lemon juice to aid digestion and keep you hydrated.

Breakfast: Oats with some nuts or blueberries for extra flavor. Remember that your oats shouldn't contain any sugar because that's what you're removing today.

Brunch: Eat a snack of full fat cultured or organic yogurt with half a banana.

Lunch: Eat a four-ounce piece of chicken or turkey and freshly cooked spinach. Use lemon juice and olive oil for dressing. You can still add some pita bread to this because you're still eating carbohydrates.

Afternoon Snack: Slice a green apple and top it with cottage cheese.

Dinner: Fry a piece of wild seafood of choice in garlic butter. Your sides can include a smaller portion of brown rice and broccoli that's been steamed and placed in the pan to absorb the fatty sauces from your fish.

Day two is when I want you to remove bread and starches. Your water intake should remain steady and you can use protein and fat to replace your starchy carbohydrates. Stop eating potatoes, pasta, and oats now too.

Breakfast: Why not have an English style breakfast that's high in protein and fat? Three strips of bacon, two eggs, one fried tomato, and mushrooms to compensate for your loss of toast.

Brunch: Thickly sliced cucumber with almond butter or organic peanut butter spread over it.

Lunch: A piece of fatty rump steak, grilled in olive oil with garlic and Himalayan salt. You can include a side salad of assorted lettuce, chickpeas, feta cheese, and tomato topped with olive oil and organic balsamic vinegar.

Afternoon snack: An avocado Ritz with shrimp.

Dinner: Eat a grilled chicken quarter with the skin on. You can create a lemon butter for this and add some chilies to your butter. Add carrots and peas as a side.

Day three is when I want you to use the vegetable products to replace your usual carbohydrate fetishes. Keep your water intake steady and add two cups of green tea to your diet today.

Breakfast: Make a three-egg omelet and include cottage cheese, onions, and mushrooms as a filling.

Brunch: Eat a full-fat organic yogurt with a handful of strawberries.

Lunch: Use a cauliflower pizza crust to create a delectable pizza with toppings that include beef strips, mushrooms, jalapeno, and homemade tomato salsa base. I'll elaborate on recipes for these in the next chapter.

Afternoon snack: Eat two boiled eggs that contain avocado and balsamic drizzle as a stuffing.

Dinner: Make a freshly ground beef stroganoff with zucchini as your pasta replacement. Use coconut cream instead of regular cream and slice the zucchini in shavings that resemble fettuccine pasta. You can flavor this with ground peppercorns and Himalayan salt.

Do you notice how the ingredients and changes have happened slowly over the three days? You can focus on specific quantities with portion size and carbohydrate intake after the three days are over.

Five Day Plan

This is a longer detox and introduces your body even slower to the changes. Each day will remove certain toxins by introducing a new healthy factor to your diet before the bad foods are removed. Portion sizes don't matter too much during the detox either and you can just focus on adding simple ingredients daily.

Day one will be your introduction to the higher fat content in your diet. Start by introducing yourself to omega-3 butter and oils, as well as a protein with higher healthy fat content such as fatty fish, rump steak, and chicken that still contains skin.

Day two is when you implement a change in protein intake. Increase your protein with boiled eggs, dairy, chicken, turkey, seafood, beef, lamb, organ meat, and even pork.

Day three is when you'll add the vegetable that you'll be using in the diet. Consider any vegetables that contain the least amounts of carbohydrates. These include spinach, cauliflower, bell peppers, and a few more.

Day four is when you start restricting your refined sugars. It's time to pack away all the sweet additives you've been hiding in the closet and stop snacking on any product that contains added sugars. This includes your snack bars, chocolate, toffees, chewing gum, and even the sugar you place in your coffee. Use stevia from this point onwards.

Day five is the final removal of carbohydrates in general. Throw your bread, pasta, potatoes, and rice in the garbage. Forget about using crackers for snacks and reduce your overall carb intake.

Once again, you've detoxed in steps that were easy to follow. You can adjust portions and record exact carbs from day six onwards.

Seven and Ten Day Plans

I would advise that you follow a longer plan, depending on the amount of damage your compulsive eating behavior has had on you. I'm sure you're getting the rhythm I'm trying to share with you because I am totally against any form of prolonged fasting before you diet. I've suffered failure before I even started because of the infamous egg fast and juice fast. Stay away from them because your body will go into devastating withdrawal from carbohydrates. I speak from experience.

After the five-day plan, there come the seven and ten-day detoxes. Quite frankly, you can adjust the five-day detox to suit either. If you're considering the seven-day detox, you can follow the first three days of your five-day strategy and use days four and five twice. When it comes to the ten-day detox, you can use each of the five-day plans twice over. I required a longer detox after my many attempts at the fasting conundrum of failures I attempted.

I'll share the foods you should and shouldn't eat in the next chapter and you can add one food group at a time before you eradicate the no-go food groups. This is the only proper technique to introduce your body to a diet before you charge at the frontline. While you're slowly depriving your body of the negative nutrients it's used to, your body's system will shift and prepare for the new foods slowly with each new one you introduce.

The Master Cleanse

This is a slightly more drastic cleanse and I don't advise it for people who fear the sound of it alone. You can consider this an intermittent fast which only lasts 24 hours before the food is reintroduced into your system. If you start your detox at eight in the morning, you should end it at eight the following morning. I agree that fasting isn't suitable for obese individuals, but a short spurt can't harm you if you have the guts to go through with it (Scrivens, n.d.). A short fasting stint can lower your insulin, increase metabolism, lower blood pressure, enhance your control of cravings, increase brain activity, and give your weight loss a jump start.

Day one: This is the 24-hour strict fasting period. You need to drink lemon water while you're fasting. You can also include green tea or apple cider vinegar diluted in water. Make this by adding one-part vinegar to five parts of warm water. As for coffee addicts, you can moderately consume black, sugarless coffee.

Day two: This is a vegetable fast. You get to enjoy an array of vegetables in any form you like as long as you eat these vegetables in four or five meals throughout the day. The veggies you're allowed to eat are cauliflower, bell peppers, celery, beets, asparagus, broccoli, Brussels sprouts, kale, mushrooms, spinach, and onions. Add tomato as the only fruit allowed today. Please do enjoy experimenting with these ingredients. The only rule is that you're only allowed to consume vegetables. This will replenish many of the nutrients you've lost in your previous fast.

Day three: You can bring the protein back now and should aim for two meals with protein throughout the day. You can add any proteins listed in the final chapter to your vegetables from the previous day. There you have it. I may be against fasting personally, but I provided you with one technique that doesn't deprive your body until it submits to cravings and emotional turmoil.

Chapter 10: The Nurturing Diet

Finally, you've reached the part you dreaded before you read this book. However, now you're revving to go because the knowledge you've gained has given you a new perspective. You'll start by eliminating what you shouldn't consume and plan your diet so that you may start. I'll even give some great recipes to help you change your life for good and remove any misconceptions about dieting being no fun.

Healthy Vs. Unhealthy Foods

I've mentioned foods and food groups throughout the book; however, now I want to place them in categories that are easy to understand and add a table with daily values you can aim for once you find your rhythm. I've added a conversion table for your convenience. A tablespoon is marked as Tbsp., a teaspoon is marked as Tsp., a fluid ounce is marked as fluid oz., and grams are marked as g throughout this chapter.

Cups	Tbsp.	Tsp.	Fluid oz.	Butter (g)	Nuts (g)
1/4	4	12	2	60	38
1/2	8	24	4	120	75
3/4	12	36	6	180	113
1	16	48	8	240	150
1 1/2	24	72	12		
2	32	96	16		

Healthy Fat and Protein Sources

Let's begin with the fat groups because this should consist of 70% of your diet. I'll include protein values for each item so that you can accurately create your diet plan. Your protein intake should consist of a 20% daily intake. Some items will contain carbohydrate values as well and these you should watch out for. You need to consume tons of healthy omega-3 and moderate unsaturated fats. You want to steer clear of any trans fatty acids, saturated fats, and keep your carbs low. The list of ingredients and substances below add to your healthy fats and proteins required in this diet.

FOOD GROUP / SIZE	DESCRIPTION	FAT (g)	PROTEIN (g)	CARBS (g)
MEAT (4 oz.)	ORGANIC BEEF	12	27	0
	WILD DUCK	60	8	0
	PORK	60	10,8	0
	WILD TURKEY	2.4	25.6	0
	CHORIZO SAUSAGE	100	56	4.4
SEAFOOD / FISH (4 oz.)	WILD SALMON	6.8	24.4	0
	MACKEREL	2.4	23.2	0
	HERRING	10.4	20.4	0
	FISH OIL SARDINES	112	0	0
	FRESH TUNA	5.6	26.4	0
	RAINBOW TROUT	7.2	22.8	0
	PERCH	1.2	22	0
	ALASKAN POLLOCK	0.8	19.6	0
	OYSTERS	19.6	92	0
	ANCHOVIES	19.2	80	0
BUTTER (1 Tbsp.)	UNSALTED ORGANIC BUTTER	11	0	0
	NATURAL GHEE	14	0	0
OIL (1 Tbsp.)	EXTRA VIRGIN OLIVE OIL	13.5	0	0
	AVOCADO OIL	14	0	0
	CANOLA OIL	14	0	0
	COCONUT OIL	13	0	0
	PEANUT OIL	13.5	0	0
DAIRY (1 cup)	FULL CREAM WHOLE MILK	8.1	7.9	12
	HEAVY WHIPPING CREAM	36	2.8	2.8
	FULL FAT GREEK YOGHURT	5	9	4
	KEFIR / CULTURED MILK	1	3.8	4.8
SPREADS/DIPS (1 Tbsp.)	OMEGA-3 PEANUT BUTTER	8.7	3.9	2.7
	UNSALTED ALMOND BUTTER	8.9	3.4	3
	AVOCADO (1 cup)	23	5.1	18
EGGS SINGLE	WHOLE ORGANIC EGG YOLK	4.5	2.7	0.6
	EXTRA LARGE ORGANIC EGG	5.3	7	0.3
VEGETARIAN	EDAMAME (1 cup)	8.1	18	14
	TOFU (1 oz.)	8.6	15	2.8
SNACK	BEEF JERKY (1 oz.)	7.3	9.4	3.1

FOOD GROUP / SIZE	DESCRIPTION	FAT (g)	PROTEIN (g)	CARBS (g)
CHEESE (1 oz.)	PLAIN CREAM	4.7	2.2	1.9
	PLAIN COTTAGE	1.2	3.2	1
	GOAT'S MILK	6	5.3	0
	PARMESAN	7.1	10	0.9
	EDAM	8.1	7.1	0.4
	BRIE	7.9	5.9	0
	LOW-SODIUM FETA	6.1	4	1.1
	BLUE	8.2	6.1	0.7
	GOUDA	7.8	7.1	0.6
	CHEDDAR	9.4	6.5	1
NUTS (1 oz.)	WALNUTS	18	4.3	3.9
	ALMONDS	14	6	6.1
	PISTACHIOS	13	5.7	7.7
	MACADAMIAS	21	2.2	3.9
	BRAZIL NUTS	19	4.1	3.3
	PECAN	20	2.6	3.9
SEEDS (1 Tbsp.)	FLAXSEEDS	4.3	1.9	3
	CHIA	2.4	1.3	3.4
	HEMP	5	3	0.8
	SESAME	4.5	1.6	2.1
	PUMPKIN	4.6	2.8	1
	SUNFLOWER	5	2	2
POWDER (1 Tbsp.)	SPIRULINA	0.5	4	1.7
VEGETABLES (1 cup)	BROCCOLI	0	2.6	6
	ASPARAGUS	0	3	5

Carbohydrate Replacement Sources

Your carbs are only allowed to amount to 10% of your daily intake, and you can use these products that contain little to no carbs to satisfy your needs.

Stevia contains no additives and is an herbal extract. One packet or five drops contains 1g of carbs. Spices that contain little to no carbs and minimal fat include cumin, turmeric, chili powder, sea salt, Himalayan salt crystals, black whole peppercorns, oregano, cilantro, thyme, basil, garlic powder, onion powder, and cayenne pepper.

The carbs you can count in your diet are mainly in your vegetables and fruits. I've calculated the carbs per cup of chopped vegetables. I'm not going to repeat the vegetables from the previous section, and I'll focus on the carbs in each of them only because the protein and fat are virtually non-existent. Please be advised that fruit is high in carbohydrates and therefore I'll use ½ cup measurements.

FOOD GROUP / SIZE	DESCRIPTION	CARBS (g)
VEGETABLES (1 cup)	BELL PEPPERS	6.9
	MUSHROOMS	2.3
	ZUCCHINI	0.5
	CHILLIES	3.6
	SPINACH	1.1
	GREEN BEANS	7
	CAULIFLOWER	5.3
	LETTUCE	1
	KALE	0.9
	CUCUMBERS	2.9
	BRUSSEL SPROUTS	7.9
	BUTTERNUT SQUASH	16
	CARROTS	12
	CELERY	3
	RADISHES	3.9
	ONIONS	15
	EGGPLANT	4.8
	CABBAGE	5.2
GOOD FRUIT (1/2 cup)	TOMATOES	2.5
	LEMON JUICE	2.1
OTHER FRUIT (1/2 cup)	WATERMELON	5.5
	BLUEBERRIES	10.5
	STRAWBERRIES	6.5
	BLACKBERRIES	7
	RASPBERRIES	7.5
	GREEN / PINK APPLES	8.5
	HONEYDEW MELON	7.5
	BANANA	17
	YELLOW PEACH	7.5

Should you wish to use a calculator to see the value of any ingredient you want to use in your meals, you can use the helpful calculator found at www.nutritionvalue.org/nutritioncalculator.php. This calculator provides you with an option to add ingredients to a meal so that you can assess the overall valuation of what you're about to eat.

Keep your diary filled with nutritional value and remember to count the carbs rather than calories.

Additional Safe Products

Please remember to read the labels of each and rather look for recipes online to make your own sauces at home. Some sauces you may use in moderation to spice things up are:

- Dijon mustard.
- Tomato paste.
- Pesto.
- Italian low carb mayonnaise.
- Guacamole.
- Salsa.
- Low carb blue cheese dressing.
- Low carb and low sodium balsamic vinegar.

Some snack ideas for low carb dieters include:

- Celery, cucumber, or bell pepper sticks with a low carb cream cheese dip or peanut butter.
- All the nuts listed in the previous categories.
- Your choice of berries with a low carb whipping cream.
- Onion rings.

- Egg muffins made with cheese to bind the ingredients.
- Gouda cheese wrapped in bacon.
- Kale chips.

The Untouchables of a Low Carb Diet

This is a list of food I've prepared to help you understand what you can't touch. I won't even bother adding values to them because you should avoid them if you want to succeed.

- White, brown, and whole wheat bread.
- Tortillas, tacos, and bagels.
- Processed cold meats.
- Raisins, dates, mangoes.
- Corn, potatoes, and sweet potato.
- Pasta in general.
- Cereals including oats, whole grain, and sugary cereals.
- Alcohol is a no go.
- Any sweetened or fruit-flavored yogurt.
- Fruit juice.
- Low fat or fat-free salad dressing.
- Beans and legumes should be kept to a minimum.
- All sugar forms including honey.
- Potato or corn chips and crackers.
- Gluten-free sweet or baked treats.
- Diet "sugar-free" products that contain aspartame.

The Diet Plan

Now you have a breakdown of the ingredients you may use. There's a larger variety than you expected and if you wish to learn more about any product, you can use the calculator I shared with you. I'm going to provide you with a seven-day plan that can be customized with your own choices, as long as they remain within the rules. Portion sizes may be larger at first but as soon as you cope better, you can decrease them to the portions I've included here. I'm going to give you a rough list of ingredients for each meal and not the recipe itself because I want you to experiment. I'll share some of my favorite recipes with you in the next section, which you may use to add to your diet. This plan will contain three meals and two light snacks per day.

Day One

Breakfast: Two scrambled eggs on some lettuce with a topping of half a cup of avocado.

Snack: Half an ounce of almonds.

Lunch: Butter grilled four-ounce salmon on top of a fresh spinach salad.

Snack: Celery sticks with a quarter cup of guacamole.

Dinner: A six-ounce pork neck steak with one cup of cauliflower mash and half a cup of apple and cabbage slaw.

Day Two

Breakfast: Two hard-boiled eggs with half a cup of white button mushrooms and a cup of bulletproof coffee.

Snack: One small cup of Greek yogurt with five crushed macadamia nuts, cocoa powder, and stevia.

Lunch: Two ounces of tuna shredded and added to a green salad with tomatoes, lettuce, cucumber, and feta cheese. The salad shouldn't amount to more than one and a half cups.

Snack: Five thickly sliced gouda strips wrapped in ghee dried bacon.

Dinner: Four ounces of minced pork meatballs on a bed of zucchini spaghetti.

Day Three

Breakfast: A two-egg omelet with half an ounce of cream cheese, a sprinkle of bacon bits, and fresh chives.

Snack: A quarter ounce of carrot sticks with homemade salsa dip.

Lunch: Vegetable soup made with one and a half cups of chopped peppers, chilies, eggplant, and spinach. Add two ounces of ground organic beef.

Snack: Half an ounce of pecan nuts.

Dinner: A skin-on chicken quarter roasted with garlic butter. Add a side of half a cup sautéed mushrooms and six storks of butter asparagus.

Day Four

Breakfast: A smoothie that combines half a cup of almond milk, half an ounce of goat's milk cheese, one finely diced red chili pepper, cilantro, and a drop of basil pesto. Trust me, this tastes great.

Snack: Six thickly sliced Edam slices topped with half an ounce of cottage cheese and fresh oregano.

Lunch: Three ounces of sliced beef rump steak, a quarter cup of mixed sliced bell peppers, a quarter cup of cucumbers sliced, a quarter cup of guacamole, and cream cheese wrapped in lettuce.

Snack: A half a cup of snack salsa with peppers, cucumbers, and blocks of cheddar.

Dinner: A four-ounce mackerel smothered in lemon butter and grilled. Add a side of cabbage and onion rings sautéed to perfection.

Day Five

Breakfast: Two fried eggs and two strips of bacon with a half a cup of green salad.

Snack: A cup of kefir.

Lunch: A turkey burger with no buns. Use lettuce, tomato, low-carb mayonnaise, butter, and a thick slice of gouda.

Snack: Three celery sticks with two tablespoons of almond butter.

Dinner: Two oven grilled lamb chops with a side of cheesy broccoli.

Day Six

Breakfast: An avocado Ritz with creamy and spicy shrimp.

Snack: Half an ounce of beef jerky.

Lunch: Homemade salmon sushi rolls made with rice-free ingredients. You can use three ounces of salmon, seaweed, avocado, and a homemade chili dip.

Snack: A small pack of kale chips.

Dinner: Cauliflower rice with garlic and lemon juice topped with a four-ounce fatty beef sirloin.

Day Seven

Breakfast: A lettuce wrap with two scrambled eggs, a quarter cup of bacon, half an ounce of cottage cheese, half a cup of bell peppers, and a quarter cup of raw mushrooms.

Snack: A quarter cup of strawberries with half an ounce of heavy whipping cream.

Lunch: Two ounces of sliced chorizo sausage with a creamy, cheesy, broccoli and cauliflower roasted combo.

Snack: Turkey jerky with half an apple sliced.

Dinner: Four ounces of fresh oysters with a creamy garlic butter dip on the side. Eat this with a fresh salad made of lettuce, tomato, bell peppers, cucumbers, and blue cheese. Your salad shouldn't exceed one and a half cups.

Feel free to make the changes you desire, but as you can see you won't go hungry as long as you use ingredients you need. Measure your carbs for every meal you plan.

The Best Recipes to Enhance Your Life

There are some recipes I couldn't have survived without. They aren't all full recipes but rather additives to your meal plan to make your meals less boring. Keep in mind that these recipes are my variations and the nutritional value was worked out according to the quantities I used. I've added a simple conversion table to make it easier for you so that we can work with cups, teaspoons (Tsp), and tablespoons (Tbsp) for the most part. I'll use ounces (oz.) and pounds (lbs) if necessary.

Homemade Ranch Dressing

Nutritional Information: 5.5g fat, 0.4g protein, 0.8g carbs.

Time: 20 minutes

Serving Size: 2 Tbsp

Ingredients:
- ½ cup heavy cream
- ½ cup sour cream
- ½ cup low carb mayonnaise
- ½ Tsp onion powder
- 1 Tsp finely crushed fresh garlic
- ½ Tsp peppercorns and sea salt crystals crushed
- 1 ½ Tsp chives
- 1 ½ Tsp tarragon
- 1 to 1 ½ tbsp lemon juice

Directions:
1. Combine all the spices and herbs.
2. Do the same with the creams and add lemon juice.
3. Mix the ingredients in a large bowl and stir.
4. Refrigerate overnight.

Guacamole

Nutritional Information: 8g fat, 1g protein, 2g carbs.

Time: 15 minutes

Serving size: 2 Tbsp

Ingredients:
- 3 Tbsp diced cilantro
- Freshly ground Himalayan salt crystals to taste

- 1 chopped jalapeno with seeds
- 1 whole red onion diced
- ½ a lemon juice freshly squeezed
- ¼ cup finely diced tomato
- 3 large or 4 medium avocados

Directions:
1. Peel the avocados and remove the pits.
2. Use a fork to mash the avocado in a medium bowl.
3. Add lemon juice ensuring an even spread. You can use more if you need.
4. Fold the remaining ingredients into the smooth avocado mash.
5. Mix well and taste to test the seasoning.

Spicy Salsa

Nutritional Information: 1g protein and 7g carbs.

Time: 10 minutes

Serving size: ¼ cup

Ingredients:
- 2 cups finely chopped tomatoes
- ½ cup diced chilies. The chili heat can be altered according to your preference
- 1 cup of pure tomato juice with no additives. It's best to juice your own tomatoes
- ½ cup diced onion
- 1 jalapeno with or without seeds
- ¼ cup diced bell peppers

- 1 clove of freshly minced garlic
- ½ cup fresh cilantro
- ½ tsp cumin
- Freshly ground sea salt to taste
- 1 Tbsp lemon juice

Directions:

1. Use a blender or a food processor to blend all the ingredients well.
2. Place the salsa in an airtight container.
3. Keep for up to five days in the fridge.

Creamy Dip for All Occasions

Nutritional Information: 9.1g fat, 1.6g protein, and 0.5g carbs.

Time: 2 minutes

Serving Size: 1 tbsp per serving

Ingredients:
- 1 ¼ cup of cream cheese
- ¼ Tsp garlic powder
- ¼ Tsp onion powder
- ½ Tsp basil
- ½ Tsp cilantro
- 1 Tbsp chives
- Freshly ground peppercorns to taste
- ½ Tsp ground Himalayan salt crystals

Directions:

1. Place all your ingredients in a medium bowl.
2. Use a fork to mix them well.
3. Keep refrigerated.

Feel free to change the spices on this one to suit your taste.

Homemade Mayonnaise

Nutritional Information: 57g fat, 1g protein, and 0.2g carbs.

Time: 10 minutes

Serving size: 2 Tbsp

Ingredients:

- 1 cup extra virgin olive oil
- 1 Tsp room temperature Dijon mustard
- 1 Tsp white wine vinegar
- 1 extra-large room temperature egg yolk
- Freshly ground pepper and salt to taste
- Add 1 Tsp of a spice or herb. Herbs of choice: cilantro, basil, chives, paprika, cayenne pepper

Directions:

1. Use a hand blender to mix the egg and mustard into a paste.
2. Gradually add the oil in a slow stream to your mix while continuing to blend.
3. Blend until mixture thickens to resemble mayonnaise.
4. Add the white wine vinegar and seasoning.
5. Blend some more until the mixture begins to set.
6. Refrigerate the mayonnaise overnight.

Cauliflower Pizza Base

Nutritional Information: 7g fat, 11g protein, and 4g of carbs.

Time: 35 minutes

Serving Size: 2 slices

Ingredients:

- 4 cups of cauliflower florets
- 1 large egg
- ¼ Tsp onion powder
- ½ Tsp garlic powder
- ½ cup grated parmesan
- ½ cup grated feta
- 1 pinch of freshly ground salt crystals & peppercorns

Directions:

1. Preheat your oven to 380°Fahrenheit.
2. Use a hand blender or food processor to create fine cauliflower pieces.
3. Place your cauliflower rice florets in the oven for five minutes to dry roast.
4. Add your seasoning and cheese to the cauliflower and return to the oven until the cheese melts.
5. Remove it from the oven and stir your egg in.
6. Prepare an oven pan with parchment paper and olive or avocado oil spray.
7. Shape your dough into a pizza shape and give the edges a little crust.
8. Bake this base for 20 minutes alone and then you can add toppings of your choice.

Zucchini Spaghetti

Nutritional Information: 14g fat, 3g protein, and 7.8g carbs.

Time: 15 minutes

Serving Size: 1 portion

Ingredients:
- 3 large zucchinis
- ¼ cup of water
- 2 Tbsp peanut oil
- ½ clove of fresh garlic
- Freshly ground Himalayan salt and black pepper to taste

Directions:
1. Peel the zucchinis before you use a julienne slicer to make them look like spaghetti strands.
2. Don't use the seeds.
3. Add garlic and oil to a hot skillet and fry the zucchini strips for 1 minute.
4. Add your water and cook for five to six minutes until the veggie is soft.
5. Season to your liking.

Low Carb Power Protein Shake

Nutritional Information: 2.7g fat, 16.7g protein, and 2.4g carbs.

Time: 15 minutes

Serving size: 1 cup

Ingredients:
- ½ cup collagen powder
- 1/5 cup stevia

- 2 Tbsp freshly ground chia seeds
- ¼ cup natural cocoa powder
- 1 pinch of sea salt
- 3 cups almond or coconut milk
- 3 cups of water

Directions:
1. Mix the dry ingredients well.
2. Mix the water and milk separately.
3. Add your dry ingredients gradually to the liquid in a blender.
4. Refrigerate for up to two days.

A Low Carb Sweet Treat

Nutritional Information: 2.2g fat, 9g carbs, 1.3g protein.

Time: 5 minutes

Serving Size: 1 portion

Ingredients:
- ½ cup of coconut yogurt
- ¼ cup crushed almonds
- ½ cup chopped strawberries
- You can use ¼ cup Greek yogurt combined with a ¼ cup coconut cream if you can't find coconut yogurt

Directions:
1. Drop a few teaspoons of yogurt in the bottom of a short glass.
2. Top this with a pinch of crushed almonds.
3. Add half of your strawberries.

4. Add some more yogurt and another pinch of almonds.
5. Add your remaining strawberries and the last of your yogurt.
6. Sprinkle with the remaining almonds.
7. Place your homemade parfait in the fridge to cool off.

This is another recipe that can use many variations of sprinkles and layers. Just keep your carb count in check throughout your experiments.

There you go. I've given you a few recipes to spruce up the boring idea of dieting.

Chapter 11: Bonus Examples

I would like to provide you with examples of two descriptions I've provided without showing you how they look. The first will be a CBT style journal in which you can keep track of your emotional wellbeing, automatic thoughts, behaviors, and possible alternatives. This journal will help you refer back to any issues that you would like to reassess.

SITUATION	THOUGHT	FEELING	EVIDENCE FOR	EVIDENCE AGAINST	ALTERNATIVE THOUGHT	RECHECK
Adam cancelled dinner	Adam is ashamed of my obesity	Anger (80%) Hurt (90%)	Adam never cancels plans	He told me that he had flu 2 days ago	Adam may still be sick and never meant to hurt me	Anger (30%) Hurt (25%)

I've spoken briefly about the journal before, but you can see in the first column, you record any situation that upsets you, including external experiences. The second column records your immediate thought and the third column is your direct emotions after, including a percentage. The fourth and fifth columns allow you to think it through again before the sixth column records your new thought after investigation. The final column will provide you with a percentage recheck on your feelings. Keep this journal and watch as the repetitive behavior grabs hold when you pause to think about every situation thoroughly. You're given the chance to challenge your thoughts this way.

The final example I want to share is a copy of my food diary. I use one page every three days and I have files filled with these papers already. It helps me keep track of what I eat, and I've discussed the diary in previous chapters.

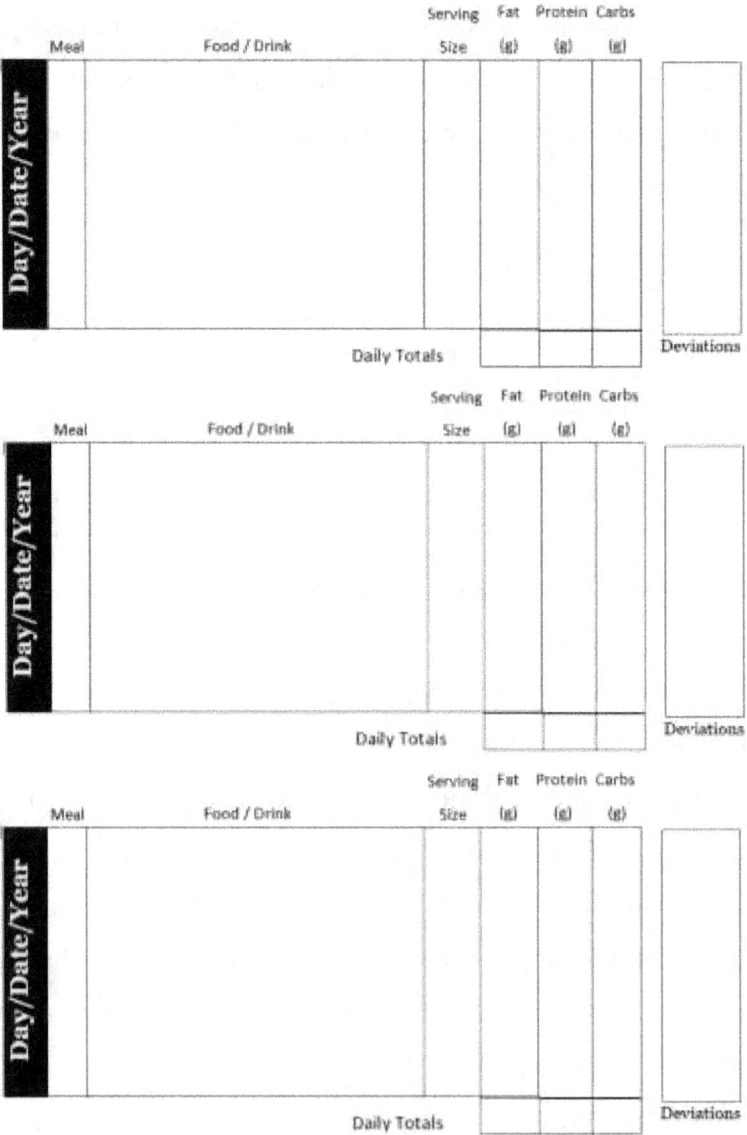

Conclusion

Michael Phelps once said, "There will be obstacles. There will be doubters. There will be mistakes. But with hard work, there are no limits." After everything you've been through, everything you've overcome, I can tell you something: You make me proud as hell.

Obstacles were placed in your path and you had no idea how to overcome them. Your weight reached a stage that made you feel hurt and disappointed in yourself. The fact that you never gave up shifts disappointment to well-deserved pride. The physical ailments that troubled you in the past can be diminished now and controlled acceptably. Down with cholesterol! Down with heart palpitations! Down with irregular menstrual cycles! Hell, the bedsores that made you so uncomfortable have bitten the dust now.

The shameful notions that have passed through your mind every day can kiss your ass now. The same buttocks that will fit back into the clothes you ultimately desire when you burn your fat with a metaphorical flamethrower. You're free from guilt and anger, not to mention the depressing mood that sat on your shoulders like a globe. You can finally flick the devil off your shoulder when he tries to convince you to take a bite of that scrumptious looking glazed donut. Your impulsive urges that controlled your thoughts and behavior can take a back seat when you apply the numerous techniques you've gathered. There's no need to stand in front of the mirror and obsess over your image as the tears roll down your cheeks anymore.

You will overcome the physical challenges that kept you indoors for so long and be a part of the hobbies and interests that you've always wished for. Think about wanting to travel and no longer having to pay additional charges for extra space. You're free to travel the world now and face any fears that hindered you before. Create a bucket list for the death of your fat and the only difference is that this list will relate to goals. You can even add skydiving to your list. There's nothing to hold you back from living the life you want.

How can any diet match science combined with techniques practiced for thousands of years? I've provided you with the fuel to remove every contributor to your disorder and not just food. The best is that you can retain food that you desire by replacing your current choices with food that helps you. The variety of options you're presented allows you to soothe insatiable desires for food that's created the person you are now. There's a great chance that this will be changed permanently as long as you believe in yourself. I've shared all the knowledge that helped me on my journey, and nothing can convince me it won't work for you. I've got three eating disorders that stain my historical timeline and for years; they've left no new blotches. If I can do it so can you. You should never feel alone again because once you know how the modern world has created obesity and eating disorders, among other factors, you can see why this "disease" has spread across every continent. Eating disorders have no preference and that harmful arrow never missed me; neither did it fly past you.

The practical methods provided in this book have opened your mental, physical, and emotional being to a whole new world. Suddenly, exercise has a new meaning because it doesn't only define physical activity. The word challenge has shifted into something that you desire and changing every part of your life with simple advice encourages you to welcome this challenge. Don't be anything less than you want to be. Change your diet, your mind, your wellbeing, and your future by stepping out of your comfort zone and knocking the ball for a home run. After all, it costs you nothing more than your previous life did.

I would love to keep tabs on the people I've assisted, and if you find clarity, resolution, and promise in my book, you're welcome to leave a review on Amazon to encourage other people to follow suit.

My final word is that you believe in yourself because I know you can change and I'm rooting for you every step of the way.

References

101 Low Carb Weight Loss Tips from the Experts. (n.d.). Retrieved from https://cutthekillercarbs.com/weight-loss-tips/101-low-carb-weight-loss-tips-from-the-experts/

Ackerman, C.E. (2019). 25 CBT Techniques and Worksheets for Cognitive Behavioral Therapy. Retrieved from https://positivepsychology.com/cbt-cognitive-behavioral-therapy-techniques-worksheets/

Aggarwal, P. (2014). Learn Self Hypnosis to Reprogram Your Subconscious Mind. Retrieved from www.udemy.com/course/learn-self-hypnosis-to-reprogram-your-subconscious-mind/

American Heart Association. (2018). American Heart Association Recommendations for Physical Activity in Adults and Kids. Retrieved from www.heart.org/en/healthy-living/fitness/fitness-basics/aha-recs-for-physical-activity-in-adults#.VnOcBTZ2TWQ

Baum, I. (2019). The 30 Best High-Protein, Low-Carb Foods, According To Nutritionists. Retrieved from www.womenshealthmag.com/food/a19976015/high-protein-low-carbohydrate-foods/

Bell, L. & Ekern, J. (2016). Mortality Rates of BED. Retrieved from www.eatingdisorderhope.com/blog/mortality-rates-of-bed

Bjarnadottir, A. (2019). Do Detox Diets and Cleanses Really Work? Retrieved from www.healthline.com/nutrition/detox-diets-101

Bjarnadottir, A. (2016). 11 Ways to Stop Cravings for Unhealthy Foods and Sugar. Retrieved from www.healthline.com/nutrition/11-ways-to-stop-food-cravings

Brennon, B. (n.d.). Bulimia: Health Risks. Retrieved from www.eatingrecoverycenter.com/conditions/bulimia/health-risks

Butler, N. & The Healthline Editorial Team. (2016). Mood Food: Can What You Eat Affect Your Happiness? Retrieved from www.healthline.com/health/mood-food-can-what-you-eat-affect-your-happiness

Camp, N. (2016). 100 Self Esteem Affirmations That Builds Self Worth. Retrieved from https://committedtomyself.com/100-self-esteem-affirmations-that-builds-self-worth/

Cherry, K. & Gans, S. (2019). Positive Reinforcement and Operant Conditioning. Retrieved from www.verywellmind.com/what-is-positive-reinforcement-2795412

Cowden, S. & Gans, S. (2019). Obsessive-Compulsive Disorder and Eating Disorders. Retrieved from www.verywellmind.com/obsessive-compulsive-disorder-and-eating-disorders-1138191

Frédérique, R.E.; Smink, D.; & Hoek, H.W. (2012). Epidemiology of Eating Disorders: Incidence, Prevalence and Mortality Rates. Retrieved from www.ncbi.nlm.nih.gov/pmc/articles/PMC3409365/

Gillihan, S. & Hampton, D. (n.d.). The Best Brain Possible. Retrieved from https://thebestbrainpossible.com/habits-brain-mental-health-therapy-cbt/

Grilo, C.M.; Masheb, R.; Wilson, G.T; Gueorguieva, R.; & White, M.A. (2011). Cognitive-Behavioral Therapy, Behavioral Weight Loss, and Sequential Treatment for Obese Patients with Binge-Eating Disorder: A Randomized Controlled Trial. Journal of Consulting and Clinical Psychology. Iss. 79, Vol. 5, P. 675-685. Retrieved from https://psycnet.apa.org/doiLanding?doi=10.1037%2Fa0025049

Hansen, K. (2013). Thoughts on Detoxing. Retrieved from https://brainoverbinge.com/thoughts-on-detoxing/

Hurst, K. (2019). How to Love Yourself and Be Confident with These 15 Self-Love Tips. Retrieved from http://www.thelawofattraction.com/love-yourself/

Karampahtis, E. (2016). What is the gastrointestinal system and how does it work? Retrieved from https://prolifestream.com/blogs/news/what-is-the-gastrointestinal-system-and-how-does-it-work

Kay, J. (2016). 7 Signs Your Friend or Loved One Might Be Struggling with an Eating Disorder. Retrieved from www.nationaleatingdisorders.org/blog/7-signs-your-friend-or-loved-one-might-be-struggling-eating-disorder

Kristeller, J.L. & Wolever, R.Q. (2011). Mindfulness-based eating awareness training for treating binge eating disorder: the conceptual foundation. Retrieved from www.ncbi.nlm.nih.gov/pubmed/21181579

Leidy, H.J.; Tang, M.; Armstrong, C.L.; Martin, C.B.; & Campbell, W.W. (2011). The effects of consuming frequent, higher protein meals on appetite and satiety during weight loss in overweight/obese men. Retrieved from www.ncbi.nlm.nih.gov/pubmed/20847729

Lewaniak, L. (2016). The Link Between Eating Disorders and Alcohol Abuse - Linda Lewaniak. Retrieved from www.eatingrecoverycenter.com/blog/2016/04/01/eating-disorders-and-alcohol-abuse-linda-lewaniak

Libby (n.d.). Top 11 Low Carb Myths. Retrieved from www.ditchthecarbs.com/top-11-low-carb-myths/

Martin, B. (2019). In-Depth: Cognitive Behavioral Therapy. Retrieved from https://psychcentral.com/lib/in-depth-cognitive-behavioral-therapy/

Medical Clinic. (2019). Whole-Body Vibration Training Protocols in Obese Individuals: A Systematic Review. Retrieved from http://www.scielo.br/scielo.php?script=sci_arttext&pid=S1517-86922019000600527&tlng=en

Mental Help.Net. (n.d.). Why Self-Esteem is Important and Its Dimensions. Retrieved from www.mentalhelp.net/self-esteem/why-its-important/

Migala, J. & Kennedy, K. (2019). Keto Diet: A Complete List of What to Eat and Avoid, Plus a 7-Day Sample Menu. Retrieved from www.everydayhealth.com/diet-nutrition/ketogenic-diet/comprehensive-ketogenic-diet-food-list-follow/

Mindful Staff. (2014). What is Mindfulness? Retrieved from www.mindful.org/what-is-mindfulness/

Mindfulness-Based Programs. Retrieved from https://link.springer.com/article/10.1007/s12671-019-01216-5

Moss, L. (2019). The 50 Weirdest Foods from Around the World. Retrieved from www.hostelworld.com/blog/the-50-weirdest-foods-from-around-the-world/

Most Obese Countries Population. (2019). Retrieved from http://worldpopulationreview.com/countries/most-obese-countries/

Murphy, R.; Straebler, S.; & Fairburn, C.G. (2010). Cognitive Behavioral Therapy for Eating Disorders. Retrieved from www.ncbi.nlm.nih.gov/pmc/articles/PMC2928448/

Newsome, T. (2016). 27 Relationship Behaviors That Might Mean You Have Low Self-Esteem. Retrieved from www.bustle.com/articles/159030-27-relationship-behaviors-that-might-mean-you-have-low-self-esteem

Nutritional Value.Org Calculator (n.d.). Retrieved from www.nutritionvalue.org/search.php?food_query=dijon+mustard

Orenstein, B.W. & Bass, P.F. (2013). 9 Ways to Mentally Prepare for Weight Loss. Retrieved from www.everydayhealth.com/weight-pictures/ways-to-mentally-prepare-for-weight-loss.aspx

Petre, A. (2019). 6 Common Types of Eating Disorders (and Their Symptoms). Retrieved from www.healthline.com/nutrition/common-eating-disorders

Rosenbloom, C. (n.d.). A sensible approach to carbs. Retrieved from www.heartandstroke.ca/articles/a-sensible-approach-to-carbs

Scrivens, P. (n.d.). 3 Day Detox Diet Plan: How to Do a Carb Detox the Easy Way. Retrieved from https://thrivestrive.com/detox-diet-plan/

Selva, J. (2019). History of Mindfulness: From East to West and Religion to Science. Retrieved from https://positivepsychology.com/history-of-mindfulness/

Shpancer, N. (2010). Overcoming Fear: The Only Way Out is Through. Retrieved from www.psychologytoday.com/us/blog/insight-therapy/201009/overcoming-fear-the-only-way-out-is-through

Spritzler, F. (2019). 14 Foods to Avoid (Or Limit) on a Low-Carb Diet. Retrieved from www.healthline.com/nutrition/14-foods-to-avoid-on-low-carb

Spritzler, F. (2018). The 21 Best Low-Carb Vegetables. Retrieved from www.healthline.com/nutrition/21-best-low-carb-vegetables

Staff of the Meadows Ranch & Ekern, J. (2018). Dealing with the Effects of Binge Eating Disorder. Retrieved from www.eatingdisorderhope.com/information/binge-eating-disorder/diagnosis-effects-consequences

Statistics and Research on Eating Disorders. (2018). Retrieved from www.nationaleatingdisorders.org/statistics-research-eating-disorders

Tarantino, O. (2016). 20 Healthy Fats to Make You Thin. Retrieved from www.eatthis.com/healthy-fats/

Teach me Physiology. (n.d.). Gluconeogenesis. Retrieved from https://teachmephysiology.com/basics/atp-production/gluconeogenesis/

The Simply Luxurious Life. (2011). Why not... Treat Your Body Like a Temple? Retrieved from www.thesimplyluxuriouslife.com/why-not-treat-your-body-like-temple/

Thompson, C.; Farrar, T.; & Bahr, M. (2020). Compulsive Eating. Retrieved from www.mirror-mirror.org/compulsive.htm

Timmons, J. & Pletcher, P. (2016). How Sedentary Obese People Can Ease into Regular Exercise. Retrieved from www.healthline.com/health/fitness-exercise/exercise-for-obese-people#1

Turgon, R.; Ruffault, A.; Juneau, C.; Blatier, C.; & Shankland, S. (2019). Eating Disorder Treatment: A Systematic Review and Meta-analysis of the Efficacy of

Vitt, C. (2017). What do Your Food Cravings Mean? Retrieved from https://deliciouslyorganic.net/what-do-your-food-cravings-mean/

Warren, M.P. (2011). Endocrine Manifestations of Eating Disorders. Retrieved from https://academic.oup.com/jcem/article/96/2/333/2709494

www.ingramcontent.com/pod-product-compliance
Lightning Source LLC
Chambersburg PA
CBHW070859080526
44589CB00013B/1124